W9-BKV-555

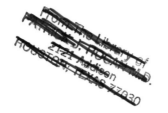

From the Library of
FARHAD SHOKOOH, M.D.
2121 Addison
Houston, Texas 77030

STATISTICS IN PRACTICE

STATISTICS IN PRACTICE

Articles published in
the *British Medical Journal*

Published by the British Medical Association
Tavistock Square, London WC1H 9JR

© British Medical Journal 1982

All rights reserved. No part of this publication may be
reproduced, stored in a retrieval system, or transmitted,
in any form or by any means, electronic, mechanical,
photocopying, recording and/or otherwise, without the
prior written permission of the publishers.

First Edition 1982
Second Impression 1984
Third Impression 1985
Fourth Impression 1988
Fifth Impression 1989
Sixth Impression 1989
Seventh Impression 1990

ISBN 0 7279 0085 4

Printed in England by The Devonshire Press, Barton Road, Torquay.
Typesetting by Bedford Typesetters Ltd, Bedford.

Preface

by the Editor *British Medical Journal*

If for medical journals the 1960s and 1970s seem likely to be remembered as the era when the importance of ethics was emphasised, the last 20 years of this century promise to be that of statistics. Not that the two are totally separate, however: as Douglas Altman has emphasised, bad statistics is bad ethics. Yet poorly designed and analysed trials are still done – and published – and, whatever the subsequent criticism, erroneous conclusions may become enshrined as the truth.

To remedy this state of affairs needs action by three groups: researchers/authors, medical statisticians, and editors of journals and their advisers. The first need to be reminded that they need statistical advice before starting a project and not at its end. The second should appreciate that most doctors are still bewildered by statistical jargon and too often react by ignoring the more important aspects of logic and correctness of argument. Thirdly, editors should be on the lookout for pitfalls and use expert statistical advisers more frequently than they do. Above all, however, their role should be as educators by reiterating the principles of statistics, telling authors where they have gone wrong, and teaching readers how to avoid mistakes.

Six years ago the *BMJ* published a series of articles by Dougal Swinscow, *Statistics at Square One*, which, collected into a book, have proved a best-seller (no fewer than 33 000 copies having been sold at the time I write). As a follow-up we commissioned two further series to illustrate the misuse of statistics in practice and how this can be put right. Both Douglas Altman and Sheila Gore have long experience of working with doctors. They have studied the quality of statistical reporting in medical journals and discovered that often it is poor. Their articles, collected here, will help those embarking on a study that will need statistics – and only a foolish researcher would start a study without thinking carefully about the statistical principles. It will also help doctors to understand and assess the results of clinical trials: some statistical understanding is a vital tool in safe and intelligent prescribing.

In retrospect, this current concern with statistics seems likely to be regarded as obvious and elementary – an attitude that will be all to the good because it will imply that statistics has become as routine a part of medical training as the need for accurate history-taking and clinical examination. Eventually, it seems likely that codes of guidelines for both authors and editors will be produced; until then, however, we hope that this book will help those who wish to understand and apply statistics to their daily work.

STEPHEN LOCK
1982

Note: Throughout this book we have followed the Vancouver convention in using p for probability, though statistical notation favours P.

Contents

STATISTICS AND ETHICS IN MEDICAL RESEARCH

DOUGLAS G ALTMAN

STATISTICS IN QUESTION

SHEILA M GORE

STATISTICS AND ETHICS IN MEDICAL RESEARCH

DOUGLAS G ALTMAN BSc

Medical statistician, Division of Computing and
Statistics, Clinical Research Centre, Harrow, Middlesex

MISUSE OF STATISTICS IS UNETHICAL

"Some people hate the very name of statistics but I find them full of beauty and interest. Whenever they are not brutalised, but delicately handled by the higher methods, and are warily interpreted, their power of dealing with complicated phenomena is extraordinary. They are the only tools by which an opening can be cut through the formidable thicket of difficulties that bars the path of those who pursue the Science of man."

FRANCIS GALTON[1]

In 1949 a divorce case was heard in which the sole evidence of adultery was that a baby was born almost 50 weeks after the husband had gone abroad on military service. To quote Barnett[2]: "The appeal judges agreed that the limit of credibility had to be drawn somewhere, but on medical evidence 349 (days), whilst improbable, was scientifically possible." So the appeal failed.

If we look at the distribution of length of gestation[3] (fig 1), which the judges apparently did not do, I think that most people would feel that the husband was hard done by. Even if we take reports of extremely long pregnancies as accurate, it is clear that, although "scientifically possible," a pregnancy lasting 349 days is an extremely unlikely occurrence. For those who believe as I do that a pregnancy of 51 weeks* exceeds the bounds of credibility, suppose it had been only 48 weeks, or 45?

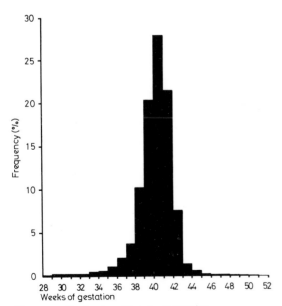

FIG 1—Frequency distribution of length of gestation.

If this case were heard now, where would *you* draw the line on the basis of figure 1?

*Using the standard convention of counting in completed weeks from the first day of the last menstrual period and assuming conception to have occurred 14 days later.

This case illustrates a failure to use statistical methods when they ought to have been used, a fairly common occurrence. Saying that an event is possible is quite different from saying that it has a probability of, say, one in 100 000. Although not an example from medical research, this case concerned essentially the same difficulty as in many more frequently encountered problems, such as defining hypertension or obesity. Everything varies; it is in trying to draw lines between good and bad, high and low, likely and unlikely, and so on, that many problems arise. Although statistics cannot answer a given question, they can often shed considerable light on the problem.

Statistics and medical ethics

So what is the relation between statistics and medical ethics? It is well appreciated that ethical considerations may affect the design of an experiment. Perhaps the most obvious examples are clinical trials—we cannot, for example, carry out controlled trials of cigarette smoking. The purpose of this series of articles is to discuss in some detail a different and much neglected aspect of the relation—how the statistical aspects affect the ethics.

Stated simply, it is unethical to carry out bad scientific experiments.[4] Statistical methods are one aspect of this. However praiseworthy a study may be from other points of view, if the statistical aspects are substandard then the research will be unethical. There are two principal reasons for this.

Firstly, the most obvious way in which a study may be deemed unethical, whether on statistical or other grounds, is the misuse of patients (or animals) and other resources. As May[5] has said: ". . . one of the most serious ethical problems in clinical research is that of placing subjects at risk of injury, discomfort, or inconvenience in experiments where there are too few subjects for valid results, too many subjects for the point to be established, or an improperly designed random or double-blind procedure."

Secondly, however, statistics affects the ethics in a much more specific way: it is unethical to publish results that are incorrect or misleading. Errors in the use of statistics may occur at all stages of an investigation, and one error can be sufficient to render the whole exercise useless. A study may have been perfectly conceived and executed, but if it is analysed incorrectly then the consequences may be as serious as for a study that was fundamentally unsound throughout.

There are many ways in which the statistical content of research may be deficient. In a fascinating and somewhat frightening recent paper, Sackett[6] identified 56 possible biases that may arise in "analytic research," over two-thirds of which related to aspects of study design and execution. Figure 2 shows how these possible biases are distributed over the stages of a research exercise. In general this distribution also reflects very well the relative seriousness of statistical errors at each stage, and indicates where there is greatest need for statistical expertise. Errors in the analysis or interpretation of results can usually be rectified if detected in time—that is, before publication—but deficiencies in the design are nearly always irremediable. The end point of the process is usually publication. Problems may

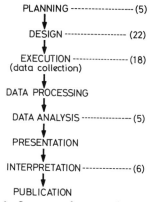

PLANNING ----------------- (5)

DESIGN ----------------- (22)

EXECUTION ---------------- (18)
(data collection)

DATA PROCESSING

DATA ANALYSIS -------------- (5)

PRESENTATION

INTERPRETATION ------------- (6)

PUBLICATION

FIG 2—Structure of a research exercise.
Explanation of numbers is given in text.

well arise when this is considered to be the most important aspect of the whole exercise, a not uncommon occurrence.

Publication

Once published, a piece of research achieves both respectability and credibility so that it is important for journals to make strenuous efforts to detect substandard research. In recent years there have been several good studies of the quality of statistics in papers in medical journals to support the idea that there is much room for improvement. For example, Schor and Karten[7] reported that, of 149 papers reporting analytical studies in several journals, only 28% were judged acceptable, 67% were deemed deficient but could be improved, and 5% were totally unsalvageable.

The editor of the journal wrote as follows:

"The study is an indirect argument for greater knowledge and appreciation of statistics by the medical author, for a reiteration on his part that the biostatistician is not a worrisome censor, but a valuable ally, and that biostatistics, far from being an unrelated mathematical science, is a discipline essential to modern medicine—a pillar in its edifice."[8]

More recent studies[9-11] have shown that there are still far too many papers being published in which the statistical analyses are incorrect. Conflicting results from similar studies can often be attributed to varying degrees of statistical competence.[12-14]

The ethical implications of publishing research containing incorrect or unfounded results or conclusions are little affected by the nature of the errors made, and are indeed much the same as the consequences of publishing spurious results. The cost in time and energy in trying to reproduce such results can be enormous.[15] Alternatively, the results may rest unchallenged for many years. Suppose a randomised controlled trial is carried out in which a conclusion is reached that the new treatment is significantly better than the previous standard treatment. The publication of such a finding may well affect patient care, and it may then be considered to be unethical to carry out further trials as one group would be denied the new treatment that was "known" to be better. Clearly, both of these consequences of publication will hold whether or not the conclusions were justified unless any deficiencies are very obvious (and many that Sackett[6] lists would not be) or if there is considerable protest. A solitary critical letter, perhaps from a

statistician, hidden away on the correspondence page is unlikely to be sufficient. Similar consequences apply in the opposite case where a treatment is incorrectly found to be ineffective.

Summary

The ethical implications of statistically substandard research may be summarised as follows:

(1) the misuse of patients by exposing them to unjustified risk and inconvenience;

(2) the misuse of resources, including the researchers' time, which could be better employed on more valuable activities; and

(3) the consequences of publishing misleading results, which may include the carrying out of unnecessary further work.

These are specific and highly undesirable outcomes. Failure to guard against these is surely as unethical as using experimental methods that offend against moral principles, such as failing to obtain fully informed consent from subjects. Surprisingly, this aspect seems to have been totally ignored by books on medical ethics.

All stages of research shown in fig 2 are vulnerable to statistical mismanagement. As an example consider one aspect of planning a study: "reading up published reports." If published papers are accepted uncritically you might be trying to verify someone else's spurious results. Remember too that authors will tend to refer to other published work that supports their arguments and ignore papers that do not.

The next few articles will illustrate some ways in which errors at different stages of a study can compromise the ethical status of the research, and discuss some ways in which they may be avoided. These will serve only as examples, since it is impossible to be comprehensive. In the final article I will consider the role of the medical journals in this context.

References

[1] Galton F. *Natural inheritance*. London: Macmillan, 1889.

[2] Barnett V. The study of outliers: purpose and model. *Applied Statistics* 1978;**27**:242-50.

[3] Chamberlain R. Birth weight and length of gestation. In: *British births 1970*. Vol 1. *The first week of life*. National Birthday Trust Fund and Royal College of Obstetricians and Gynaecologists. London: Heinemann, 1975.

[4] Denham MJ, Foster A, Tyrrell DAJ. Work of a district ethical committee. *Br Med J* 1979;ii:1042-5.

[5] May WW. The composition and function of ethical committees. *J Med Ethics* 1975;**1**:23-9.

[6] Sackett DL. Bias in analytic research. *J Chronic Dis* 1979;**32**:51-63.

[7] Schor S, Karten I. Statistical evaluation of medical journal manuscripts. *JAMA* 1966;**195**:1123-8.

[8] Anonymous. A pillar of medicine. *JAMA* 1966;**195**:1145.

[9] Gore SM, Jones IG, Rytter EC. Misuse of statistical methods: critical assessment of articles in *BMJ* from January to March 1976. *Br Med J* 1977;i:85-7.

[10] Feinstein AR. A survey of the statistical procedures in general medical journals. *Clin Pharmacol Ther* 1974;**15**:97-107.

[11] Ambroz A, Chalmers TC, Smith H, Schroeder B, Freiman JA, Shareck EP. Deficiencies of randomized control trials. *Clin Res* 1978;**26**:280A.

[12] Gifford RH, Feinstein AR. A critique of methodology in studies of anticoagulant therapy for acute myocardial infarction. *N Engl J Med* 1969;**280**:351-7.

[13] Peto R. Clinical trial methodology. *Biomedicine Special Issue* 1978;**28**: 24-36.

[14] Horwitz RI, Feinstein AR. Methodologic standards and contradictory results in case-control research. *Am J Med* 1979;**66**:556-64.

[15] Muller M. Why scientists don't cheat. *New Scientist* 1977;**74**:522-3.

STUDY DESIGN

The term "design" encompasses all the structural aspects of a study, notably the definition of the study sample, size of sample, method of treatment allocation, type of statistical design (randomised, cross-over, sequential, etc), and choice of outcome measures. The importance of this stage cannot be over-emphasised since no amount of clever analysis later will be able to compensate for major design flaws. I will consider the relation between design and ethics in observational studies and clinical trials, but I will discuss the problem of sample size in "How large a sample?" on page 6.

Observational studies

In observational studies data from a sample of individuals are used, either implicitly or explicitly, to make inferences about the population of interest, such as men aged 20-65, hypertensives, or pregnant women. For this extrapolation to be valid, it is essential that the data obtained are as representative of the population as possible.

This usually entails some type of random sampling of subjects, for which a ready-made list of the whole population of interest (a sampling frame) is needed. Such lists, however, may be out of date (electoral registers) or inaccurate (doctors' lists of patients), in which case their use can lead to misleading results. Furthermore, it is often desirable to improve the representativeness of the sample by sampling separately from different subgroups—for example, by age and sex—but this additional information may not be available.

For many populations, such as the three examples above, no sampling frame exists, so that it may be impossible to obtain a representative sample. Consider, for example, trying to select a random sample of all the preschool children in an area to estimate the prevalence of vision or hearing defects. Yet for studies such as this, which set out to estimate the prevalence or incidence of some condition, the need for a truly representative sample is particularly great—otherwise the results are of uncertain value.

Even with a good selection procedure the study may be ruined by a poor response rate. Although deemed non-invasive, such studies may entail visiting people at home, expecting them to complete and return a questionnaire, or to attend a clinic, and thus may be liable to considerable non-cooperation. Unfortunately, those who do not participate often tend to be somewhat different from those who do, both in respect of their medical condition (if this is relevant) and their social and demographic characteristics. This problem should be anticipated at the design stage, and plans made to "chase up" non-responders. It is generally advisable to keep questionnaires and other procedures short and simple to help reduce non-response. In the end, though, the response rate may largely depend on the subjects' perception of the importance of the study.

It is much less common in case-control studies to find researchers concerned about defining the subjects who will be eligible for a study, although Sackett[1] has described 22 biases that may arise at this stage. One of the most interesting is Berkson's bias, which Mainland[2] recently drew to the attention of readers of this journal. Case-control studies of hospital patients are often set up to study the relation between a specific disease and exposure to a suspected causal factor. If the hospital admission rates for exposed and unexposed cases and controls differ appreciably, then the observed association between the factor and the disease may be seriously biased (in either direction).[2 3] Indeed, the choice of control group may affect the observed association between a disease and a suspected cause. A consequence of this is that such studies may need to be supported by prospective studies.

Another of Sackett's catalogue[1] is the membership (or "self-selection") bias. He cites the example of an apparent association between lack of exercise after myocardial infarction and the increased risk of recurrent attacks. This result was found in two observational studies where exercise was taken voluntarily, but was not substantiated by a prospective randomised study.

So the major problem of all observational studies is the selection of subjects for study. This aspect must be given considerable attention at the design stage, because if the sample is not representative of the population then the results will be unreliable and of dubious worth.

Clinical trials

Whatever one's view on the best type of design, clinical trials of some sort are clearly important for new treatments. As May[4] says: "The ethical justification for such experimentation, which is outside the pure physician-patient relationship, is based on a judgment that in certain circumstances it is legitimate to put a subject at risk, with his or her consent, because of the overriding need of society for progress in combating certain diseases."

A revealing example concerns the epidemic of retrolental fibroplasia in the 1950s.[5 6] The treatment of infants with early eye changes with adrenocorticotrophic hormone was thought to be a success as there was a cure rate of 75%. A clinical trial, however, would have shown that adrenocorticotrophic hormone was ineffective since 75% of such infants return to normal without treatment. The widespread use of this treatment meant that hundreds of infants were exposed to unnecessary risk, and that discovery of the cause of the epidemic (an oxygen-rich environment) was delayed.

The debate about the ethics of clinical trials is still very active. Some authors have suggested that it is unethical *not* to carry out a clinical trial on a new treatment, whereas others believe that such trials are unethical, at least in the way they are usually conducted.

IS IT ETHICAL TO RANDOMISE?

In most clinical trials subjects are allocated to the new treatment at random, others receiving either a standard treatment or a placebo. The main ethical problem is the balancing of the welfare of the individuals in the trial against the potential benefit to future patients.

It is the random allocation of subjects that comes in for most criticism. It is argued that even if at the beginning of a trial one may not know if a treatment is effective, as the study progresses it is unethical to continue to randomise ignoring the results so far.[7] As Meier[8] has observed, however, this attitude is based on the questionable premise "that it is unethical to deny an individual any expected benefit of treatment A over treatment B, regardless of how small that benefit may be or how uncertain."

Because of the difficulty in interpreting interim results of randomised studies, two types of non-randomised study have recently found some favour and deserve a closer look.

HISTORICAL CONTROLS

Is it really necessary to have a concurrent control group when carrying out a clinical trial? Cranberg[9] has recently argued that instead one can use retrospective or "historical" controls—that is, previously collected data on patients who had received what would be the control treatment. Although widely practised, and perhaps of value in some circumstances,[10] this can be extremely risky.

The main problem of studies using historical controls is their insensitivity to secular changes, most importantly in selection criteria.[11] The worst historical data to use are other people's published results, perhaps partly because of the publication bias towards positive results. Pocock[12] gives as an example 20 studies of fluorouracil for advanced cancer of the large bowel with reported success rates ranging from 8% to 85%. But data from a previous study in the same institution may also be unreliable. Pocock reports that in 19 instances where the same treatment was used in two consecutive trials of cancer chemotherapy in one organisation the changes in death rates from one trial to the next ranged from -46% to $+24\%$, four of the differences being significant at the 2% level.

The use of historical controls is often advocated as being more ethical than using a concurrent randomised control group. The results of studies using historical controls are extremely unreliable, however, so that unless there is sound justification for their use such designs should themselves be rejected as unethical.

ADAPTIVE DESIGNS

Designs where the proportion of subjects allocated to each treatment depends on the accumulated results so far may appear preferable to randomised trials.[7] It must be realised, however, that with such designs some subjects are still allocated to the treatment that is less successful so far, not so many as with randomised studies but still essentially at random. Furthermore, because of the unequal sample sizes for the two treatments, the study may require more subjects than an equal allocation study.[8 13]

Such designs require that the result for each individual is known quickly, which is often not the case. It is implicitly assumed that there is a single outcome of interest, whereas there may be several possible methods of assessment, as well as aspects such as side effects to be considered. They are also insensitive to any secular changes during the course of the study. For these reasons, although appealing in principle, adaptive designs have rarely, if ever, been used.[8]

SEQUENTIAL DESIGNS

Sequential designs[14] may seem the best compromise in that they combine the many advantages of a randomised study with the desirable feature of taking account of the results so far in determining the length of the trial.

The main advantage over an ordinary randomised study is that the required sample size will be smaller if the treatment "effect" is larger. So the bigger the difference between treatments, the fewer subjects receive the less successful treatment.

Their main disadvantages are the same as for adaptive designs, especially the need for the results for each subject to be available quickly. Sequential designs are clearly of no value in long-term studies, where all the subjects will be recruited before any results are obtained. Nevertheless, in the right circumstances they can be useful and should probably be used more often.

CONSENT

Another problem of clinical trials is the need to obtain the "informed consent" of the subjects. In some cases this may be impossible because of the age or condition of the subjects, or because of the difficulty of explaining the scientific issues. Zelen[15] has recently proposed a new design for comparing a new treatment with a standard one that neatly avoids the problem. He proposed that, of the subjects entering a trial, half are randomly assigned to receive the standard treatment (group 1). These subjects are treated as if they were not in the trial apart from the needs of standardised assessment and record keeping. The other half (group 2) are given a choice: they are offered the new treatment B, which is under investigation, but they may have the standard treatment A if they wish. The important point is that the subjects *choose*—this is quite different from agreeing to be randomised—so that the problems associated with informed consent do not arise.

If most of the second group elect to have the new treatment B, as is quite likely, then this design will probably be more efficient overall. It is of course essential to compare group 1 with group 2, not all those undergoing treatment A with those undergoing B. In this way two randomly selected groups will be compared. There will be some loss of efficiency because group 2 is "contaminated" by a minority undergoing treatment A, but this effect is likely to be outweighed by the advantage of having virtually no refusers.

This design, which seems perfectly ethical (Zelen[15] discusses many of the issues), has two advantages over ordinary randomised trials—the ability to include all eligible subjects and the avoidance of the tricky problem of informed consent.

PLACEBOS

Too many studies compare a new treatment with a placebo rather than an existing treatment, and thus yield results that are of no practical importance. It is sometimes necessary to include placebos, but whenever possible they should be used only when there is no appropriate treatment for comparison. Invasive placebo treatment is unlikely ever to be justified.

CONCLUSIONS

There is no one best design for all clinical trials. The choice for a specific trial must depend on the seriousness of the condition being treated, the nature of the treatments, the response time, the measures of outcome, and so on. The main ethical problem is balancing the interests of the individuals in the study with those of the much larger number who may benefit in the long term. But it is also vital that the research should provide useful results, and this may often be achieved best by a randomised study (double-blind if possible). If it is thought likely that highly favourable early results or a high incidence of side effects would argue in favour of premature termination of the study, then these considerations may be built in, using a sequential design.

The ethical difficulties associated with the widespread use of a new treatment without a trial are far greater than those associated with the trial itself. The importance of good design, however, is reflected in the many examples of conflicting results that may be found in series of case-control studies of the same topic.[16] As a notable example, after 32 studies over 25 years there is still no consensus on the efficacy of anticoagulants following myocardial infarction.[11]

References

1 Sackett DL. Bias in analytic research. *J Chron Dis* 1979;**32**:51-63.
2 Mainland D. Berkson's fallacy in case-control studies. *Br Med J* 1980; **280**:330.
3 Roberts RS, Spitzer WO, Delmore T, Sackett DL. An empirical demonstration of Berkson's bias. *J Chron Dis* 1978;**31**:119-28.
4 May WW. The composition and function of ethical committees. *J Med Ethics* 1975;**1**:23-9.
5 Silverman WA. The lesson of retrolental fibroplasia. *Sci Am* 1977;**236**:100-7.
6 Herbert V. Acquiring new information while retaining old ethics. *Science* 1977;**198**:690-3.
7 Weinstein MC. Allocation of subjects in medical experiments. *N Engl J Med* 1974;**291**:1278-85.
8 Meier P. Terminating a trial—the ethical problem. *Clin Pharmacol Ther* 1979;**25**:633-40.
9 Cranberg L. Do retrospective controls make clinical trials inherently fallacious? *Br Med J* 1979;ii:1265-6.
10 Gehan EA, Freireich EJ. Non-randomized controls in cancer clinical trials. *N Engl J Med* 1974;**290**:198-204.
11 Doll R, Peto R. Randomised controlled trials and retrospective controls. *Br Med J* 1980;**280**:44.
12 Pocock SJ. Allocation of patients to treatment in clinical trials. *Biometrics* 1979;**35**:183-97.
13 Byar DP, Simon RM, Friedewald WT, *et al*. Randomized clinical trials. Perspectives on some recent ideas. *N Engl J Med* 1976;**295**:74-80.
14 Armitage P. *Sequential medical trials*. 2nd ed. Oxford: Blackwell, 1975.
15 Zelen M. A new design for randomized clinical trials. *N Engl J Med* 1979;**300**:1242-5.
16 Horwitz BI, Feinstein AR. Methodologic standards and contradictory results in case-control research. *Am J Med* 1979;**66**:556-64.

HOW LARGE A SAMPLE?

Whatever type of statistical design is used for a study, the problem of sample size must be faced. This aspect, which causes considerable difficulty for researchers, is perhaps the most common reason for consulting a statistician. There are also, however, many who give little thought to sample size, choosing the most convenient number (20, 50, 100, etc) or time period (one month, one year, etc) for their study. They, and those who approve such studies, should realise that there are important statistical and ethical implications in the choice of sample size for a study.

A study with an overlarge sample may be deemed unethical through the unnecessary involvement of extra subjects and the correspondingly increased costs. Such studies are probably rare. On the other hand, a study with a sample that is too small will be unable to detect clinically important effects. Such a study may thus be scientifically useless, and hence unethical in its use of subjects and other resources. Studies that are too small are extremely common, to judge by surveys of published research.[1] [2] The ethical implications, however, have only rarely been recognised.[3] [4]

The approach to the calculation of sample size will depend on the complexity of the study design. I will discuss it here in the context of trying to ascertain whether a new treatment is better than an existing one, since it will help if the ideas are illustrated by one of the most common types of research.

Significance tests and power

Despite their widespread use in medical research significance tests are often imperfectly understood. In particular, few medical researchers know what the power of a test is. This is perhaps because most simple books and courses on medical statistics do not discuss it in any detail, even though it is a concept fundamental to understanding significance tests. Some of the general implications, however, are well appreciated, such as the awareness that the more subjects there are, the greater the likelihood of statistical significance.

Formally, the power of a significance test is a measure of how likely that test is to produce a statistically significant result for a population difference of any given magnitude. Practically, it indicates the ability to detect a true difference of clinical importance. The power may be calculated retrospectively to see how much chance a completed study had of detecting (as significant) a clinically relevant difference. More importantly, it may be used prospectively to calculate a suitable sample size. If the smallest difference of clinical relevance can be specified we can calculate the sample size necessary to have a high probability of obtaining a statistically significant result—that is, high power—if that is the true difference. For a continuous variable, such as weight or blood pressure, it is also necessary to have a measure of the usual amount of variability. A simple example will, I hope, illustrate the relation between the sample size and the power of a test.

AN EXAMPLE

Suppose we wish to carry out a milk-feeding trial on 5-year-old children when a random half of the children are given extra milk every day for a year. We know that at this age children's height gain in 12 months has a mean of about 6 cm and a standard deviation of 2 cm. We consider that an extra increase in height in the milk group of 0·5 cm on average will be an important difference, and we want a high probability of detecting a true difference at least that large.

Figure 1 shows the power of the test for a true difference of

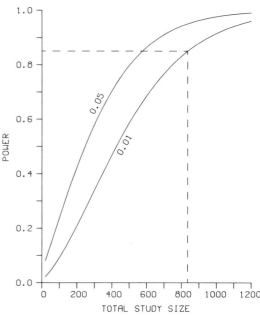

FIG 1—Relation between sample size and power to detect as significant (p<0·05 or p<0·01) a difference of 0·5 cm when standard deviation is 2 cm.

0·5 cm. The increase in power with increasing sample size is clearly seen, as is the relation with the significance level. For any given sample size the probability of obtaining a result significant at either the 5% or 1% level, given a true difference in growth of 0·5 cm, can be read off. Power of 80-90% is recommended; figure 1 shows that to achieve an 85% chance of detecting the specified difference of 0·5 cm significant at the 1% level we would need a total of about 840 children.

If we are told that we can have at most 500 children in all, what will the power be now? Figure 1 shows that the power drops from 85% to 60%. We are now more than twice as likely to miss a true difference of 0·5 cm at the 1% level, although the power is still about 80% for a test at the 5% level of significance. Alternatively, and not shown by figure 1, this size of study achieves the same power as the larger one for a difference of 0·65 cm instead of 0·5 cm. Whether or not this is thought sufficient will depend on how far one is prepared to alter one's criteria of acceptability for the sake of expediency. Although they are to some extent arbitrary, it is generally advisable to stick closely to the prestated criteria.

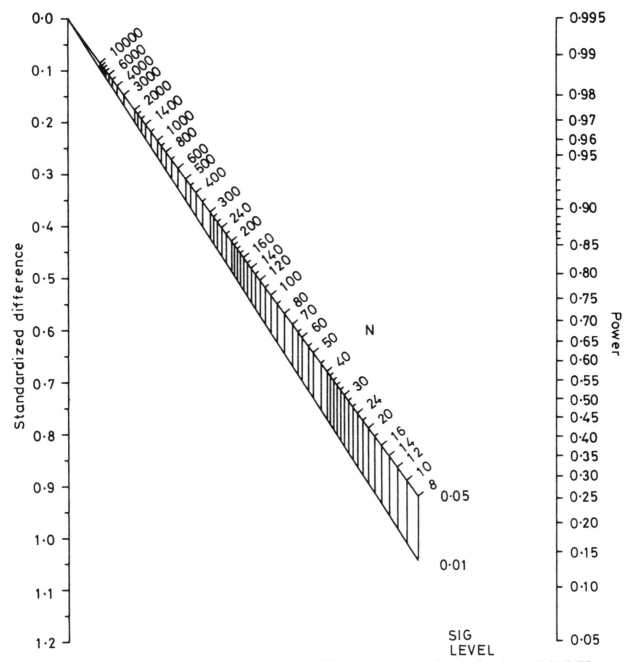

FIG 2—Nomogram for a two-sample comparison of a continuous variable, relating power, total study size, the standardised difference, and significance level.

A NEW SIMPLE METHOD

The formula on which these calculations are based is not particularly simple. Graphs are preferable, but because so many variables are concerned, a large set of graphs like figure 1 would be necessary to calculate sample size for any problem. Greater flexibility, however, is achieved by the nomogram shown in figure 2. This makes use of the standardised difference, which is equal to the postulated true difference (usually the smallest medically relevant difference) divided by the estimated standard deviation. So in the previous example the standardised difference of interest was $0.5/2.0 = 0.25$. The nomogram is appropriate for calculating power for a two-sample comparison of a continuous measurement with the same number of subjects in each group. The only restriction is the common requirement that the variable that is being measured is roughly Normally distributed.

The nomogram gives the relation between the standardised difference, the total study size, the power, and the level of significance. Given the significance level (5% or 1%),* by

*As in the example these are two-tailed significance levels.

joining with a straight line the specific values for two of the variables the required value for the other variable can easily be read off the third scale. By using this nomogram, it is both simple and quick to assess the effect on the power of varying the sample size, the effect on the required sample size of changing the difference of importance, and so on. It is easy to confirm the earlier calculations for the milk-feeding trial.

An estimate of the standard deviation should usually be available, either from previous studies or from a pilot study. Note that the nomogram is not strictly appropriate for retrospective calculations. Although it will be reasonably close for samples larger than 100, for smaller samples it will tend to overestimate the power.

QUALITATIVE DATA

For many studies the outcome measure is not continuous but qualitative—for example, where one is looking for the presence or absence of some condition or comparing survival rates. Peto *et al*[5] have discussed calculating sample size for such studies, and they emphasise the problem of getting enough subjects when either the condition is rare or the expected improvement is not large. For example, about 1600 subjects would be needed to have a power of 90% of detecting (at p <0·05) a reduction in mortality from 15% to 10%. Although the sample size will in general need to be much larger for studies including qualitative outcome measures, the logic behind the calculations is exactly the same as with continuous data, except that a prior estimate of the standard deviation is not needed. Several authors have published graphs for general use.[6-8]

OTHER TYPES OF STUDY

Sequential designs are similarly amenable to the incorporation of considerations of power at the design stage. Indeed, it is probably much more common here than for ordinary randomised studies. For these, and for more complicated designs, it may be particularly helpful to enlist the aid of a statistician when thinking about sample size.

Conclusions

The idea behind using the concept of power to calculate sample size is to maximise, so far as practicable, the chances of finding a real and important effect if it is there, and to enable us to be reasonably sure that a negative finding is strong grounds for believing that there is no important difference. The effect of the approach outlined above is to make clinical importance and statistical significance coincide, thus avoiding a common problem of interpretation.

Before embarking on a study the appropriate sample size should be calculated. If not enough subjects are available then the study should not be carried out or some additional source of subjects should be found.[5] (It should also be borne in mind that expected accession rates tend to be over-optimistic.) The calculations affecting sample size and power should be reported when publishing results. A study[2] of 172 randomised controlled trials published in the *New England Journal of Medicine* and the *Lancet* from 1973 to 1976 found that none mentioned a prior estimate of the required sample size, and none specified a clinically relevant difference that might allow calculation of the power of their study. Obviously in most of these studies such calculations were not done.

It is surprising and worrying that in such an ethically sensitive area as clinical trials so little attention has been given to an aspect that can have major ethical consequences. If the sample size is too small there is an increased risk of a false-negative finding. A recent survey[1] of 71 supposedly negative trials found that two-thirds of them had at least a 10% risk of missing a true improvement of 50%. In only one of the 71 studies was power mentioned as having been considered before carrying out the study. It is surely ethically indefensible to carry out a study with only a small chance of detecting a treatment effect unless it is a massive one, and with a consequently high probability of failure to detect an important therapeutic effect.

References

[1] Freiman JA, Chalmers TC, Smith H, Kuebler RR. The importance of beta, the type II error and sample size in the design and interpretation of the randomized control trial. *N Engl J Med* 1978;**299**:690-4.

[2] Ambroz A, Chalmers TC, Smith H, Schroeder B, Freiman JA, Shareck EP. Deficiencies of randomized control trials. *Clinical Research* 1978; **26**:280A.

[3] Newell DJ. Type II errors and ethics. *Br Med J* 1978;iv:1789.

[4] Anonymous. Controlled trials: planned deception? *Lancet* 1979;i:534-5.

[5] Peto R, Pike MC, Armitage P, *et al.* Design and analysis of randomized clinical trials requiring prolonged observation of each patient. I Introduction and design. *Br J Cancer* 1976;**34**:585-612.

[6] Aleong J, Bartlett DE. Improved graphs for calculating sample sizes when comparing two independent binomial distributions. *Biometrics* 1979;**35**:875-81.

[7] Boag JW, Haybittle JL, Fowler JF, Emery EW. The number of patients required in a clinical trial. *Br J Radiol* 1971;**44**:122-5.

[8] Mould RF. Clinical trial design in cancer. *Clin Radiol* 1979;**30**:371-81.

COLLECTING AND SCREENING DATA

Even with an impeccable design there are many ways in which a study can go wrong when the data are being collected. In general, the more complicated the design the more chance there is of the study not being carried out properly. As an example, consider this historic study. The story was related by "Student" (he of *t*-test fame):

"In the Spring of 1930 a nutritional experiment on a very large scale was carried out in the schools of Lanarkshire. For four months 10 000 schoolchildren received three-quarters of a pint of milk per day; 5000 of these got raw milk and 5000 pasteurised milk; another 10 000 children were selected as controls, and the whole 20 000 children were weighed and their height was measured at the beginning and end of the experiment."[1]

There was no power problem here! The study found that children getting extra milk gained more weight in the period than did the controls. But did the extra milk cause the extra gain? The figure is a simplified chart showing the weight changes for girls during the study. Since the two milk groups are very similar, only one is shown here. There are two striking features of this graph. The first is that the controls were in all cases heavier than those getting extra milk (they were taller too). This can be easily explained by the discovery that some of the teachers who allocated children to groups had juggled the randomisation to enable the poorer children to get the extra milk.

The second curious feature is that the observed growth rate in each group was much less than would be expected by looking at the next age group. The explanation for this is also very simple. The study began in February and ended in June, and the children were weighed on both occasions with their clothes on. The shortfall in weight increase is thus largely due to a different amount of clothing, and the smaller effect in the milk feeding group can be explained by the poorer children wearing relatively fewer clothes in winter.

It may be thought that errors such as these are really obvious, and nobody would make such mistakes nowadays. Two points may be made about the altruistic adjustment of the randomisation. Firstly, this procedure is not unknown in more recent times. Carleton *et al*[2] reported that strongly motivated doctors may upset trials by transilluminating envelopes containing the names of drugs in order to find the desired treatment. However well-intentioned, such underhand activities are by their nature likely to go undetected and can invalidate a whole study. Doctors should not agree to participate in a randomised controlled trial if they have a prior preference for one treatment. Equally, the study sample should not include subjects for which one treatment is clearly medically preferable. A trial where either of these conditions was broken would be unethical.[3]

The second point relating to the allocation of subjects to treatments is that a major reason for random allocation is to eliminate the effect of both deliberate and unconscious biases. If the groups are not selected randomly it will be impossible to know whether any observed treatment effect is genuine, as in the Lanarkshire milk trial. So what reliability can we place on the results of a study in which patients were allocated to treatments "nearly at random"?[4]

The other error in the Lanarkshire study, that of weighing children with full clothing at different times of the year, would be unlikely to be made in that form now. Errors of this sort, how-

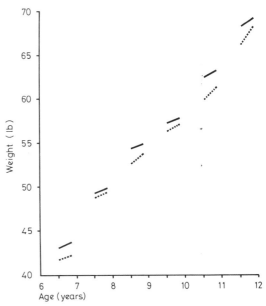

Lanarkshire milk experiment[1]: comparison of control group (———) and milk feeding group (- - - - -) showing mean weight at beginning and end of study for each yearly age group.

ever, are very easy to make, and usually occur when a source of variation is overlooked. For example, in studies looking for small differences it may be important to allow for the fact that height and blood pressure are less in the evening than in the morning, or that lung function is better in summer than in winter. Failure to allow for such things can lead to two effects being "confounded" or inseparable. So, in the milk study we cannot say how much of the difference between the groups was due to the milk, how much to the non-random allocation, and how much to the changes in clothing.

Perhaps to try to insure against this sort of problem, it is quite common for a study to collect information on anything that might possibly be of some value or interest. This seems particularly common in surveys, where one is not always investigating a specific issue but looking at a general situation. If information is being collected by questionnaire, however, then increasing the number of questions may lower the response rate, with the results being less reliable as a consequence. Further, excessive amounts of information may reduce the care given to data collection.

Data screening

Before proceeding to the analysis, some degree of data screening should be carried out. By screening is meant checking so far as is possible that the recorded values are plausible, since one can not usually know if the data are correct. Simple data sets obviously need minimal checking in comparison with studies concerning a large amount of information for each subject.

Screening the data (sometimes called cleaning or validation) entails checking that for each variable all the observations are within reasonable limits. Where feasible, each variable should also be cross-checked against other relevant information. This may show inconsistencies such as an 18-year-old woman with six children. It may also show that values that appeared odd are quite compatible with other data.

Much can be learnt from an initial close examination of the data, taking variables both one and two at a time, using histograms and scatter diagrams.[5] As well as identifying outliers, such screening of the data should disclose whether it will be necessary to transform any of the variables before analysis. It will also help to discover if any observations are missing. All of these aspects merit examination.

WHAT CAN WE DO ABOUT OUTLIERS?

Outliers are observations that are not compatible with the rest of the data. Typically there may be one or two such values in a set of data, but they can have an unduly large influence on the results of an analysis.

The first thing to do with suspicious values is to make sure that they have not been incorrectly transcribed. Any impossible values should be treated as missing data, but defining what is impossible may be very difficult. For example, how large would a value for length of gestation or maternal age be before it was considered impossible?

If an outlying observation appears correct in that the value is possible (although unlikely) and there is no evidence to suggest that it is wrongly recorded, then it should not be excluded from the analyses. It is particularly bad to remove such values purely on the grounds that they are the smallest or largest.

In small samples outlying values may have a very large influence on the results—for example, a regression line will be "pulled towards" outlying values. Ranking methods can be used, but they are generally only useful for testing hypotheses, not for the estimation of means, standard deviations, regression slopes, and so on.

WHY TRANSFORM DATA?

When analysing continuous variables (height, blood pressure, serum cholesterol, etc) it is usual to make use of a "family" of statistical analyses, including t tests, regression, and the analysis of variance, that make important assumptions about the data. Such analyses are not valid if these criteria are not met.

The best known example of this is when data display skewness instead of the required symmetric normal (Gaussian) distribution. All of the above methods have some sort of normality assumption. In such cases it is often possible to find a mathematical transformation for the data that will make the analysis valid.[5][6] By far the most common transformation used in medical research is the logarithmic transformation, needed, for example, for various biochemical measurements.[7] It is worth noting that an appropriate transformation may also have the effect of making previously suspicious values become quite reasonable.

Although it is obvious that the more nearly the underlying assumptions are met the more reliable will be the results, it is unfortunately not possible to say how far the raw data can deviate from the ideal before the results become invalid. Because of the subjective nature of this problem expert help can be particularly helpful here.

WHAT CAN WE DO ABOUT MISSING DATA?

An important distinction must be made between data that are missing through random misfortune (if some forms are mislaid, for instance) or for a reason directly or indirectly related to the study itself. Most studies have a few accidentally missing observations. These cases can usually be omitted without greatly affecting the results. It may be thought preferable to include a subject for any analyses for which data exist, only excluding him when the relevant observation is missing. This procedure can cause complications in interpretation, however, as each analysis

will be based on different subjects, and is better avoided if possible.

It is also common to have data missing through a subject's refusal to supply information or to participate in a study. The problem here is that refusers are often an atypical subgroup. In a survey it may be possible to study what is known about the refusers to see if and how they do differ from participants, and to try to estimate the effect on the results. Clearly a high refusal rate will mean that little sensible extrapolation from the sample to the population is possible.

In a randomised trial it is essential that refusers (or withdrawals) are considered as part of the group to which they were allocated.[3] A good example is given by a study[8] of the sudden infant death syndrome. High-risk infants were randomly allocated to observed and control groups, where observation consisted of increased health visitor surveillance. In the control group, where active participation did not need to be sought, there were nine unexpected deaths out of 922 infants, a rate of 9·8 per thousand. In those allocated to the "observed" group, there were two unexpected deaths out of 627 who agreed to participate (3·2 per thousand), and three out of 210 among those who refused (14·3 per thousand). This is a good example of the commonly found poor prognosis among refusers.

The purpose of a randomised trial is to be able to make comparisons between randomly allocated groups. Some trials have "observed controls" where one randomly chosen group is offered treatment while the other group is just observed. Any refusing treatment must still be considered with the treated group; otherwise the two groups will no longer be comparable (the control group do not have a chance to refuse), and it will not be possible to draw valid conclusions. Such trials are thus comparisons of different treatment policies. Alternatively trials can have "placebo controls," when only those subjects who give their informed consent to participate are randomised. Such studies give a direct comparison of treatments, although on a less representative group of subjects, but they are not always practical. The two approaches are discussed and illustrated in Meier's fascinating and very readable account of the Salk vaccine trial.[9]

The health visitor surveillance study had observed controls, so that all of those allocated to the observation group should be considered together. This gives five unexpected deaths out of 837, which is a rate of 6·0 per thousand, and is not nearly significantly different from the control group. The authors excluded the refusers from their analysis, giving a much larger apparent effect of observation (although still not statistically significant). In contrast, a recent study[10] comparing treatments for suspected myocardial infarction included withdrawals from the trial when analysing the data.

Another class of missing data is censored data—that is, values that cannot be measured. One common source is in the measurement of substances present in such low concentrations that some of the samples are below the sensitivity of the equipment being used. Another is where records are kept of the length of time for some event to happen (survival data) or the length of duration of some phenomenon, and the experiment is terminated before an answer can be obtained for all subjects. Censored data are clearly very different from missing observations, and must not be excluded from analysis; this would severely affect the results as these are the most extreme observations. Such data sets can be analysed by non-parametric (ranking) methods if only a few observations are censored at the same point. If censoring is at different values (as in survival studies) more rigorous statistical methods are necessary.

Conclusions

Problems with data collection are often the result of the failure at the design stage to anticipate unusual circumstances. This is one reason why large studies ought to have a pilot phase to try to spot any major deficiencies. It is because we cannot foresee everything that may be relevant that randomisation is so important, but it must be strictly adhered to.

The wide availability of computers and calculators has made it much easier to carry out statistical analyses. Unfortunately, they have also made it easy to produce results without ever really studying the raw data. Before embarking on analysis there is much that can be learnt from simple inspection of variables both singly and in pairs. Such screening of the data, especially graphically, as well as greatly helping to prepare the data for analysis, can also provide considerable insight into the relationships between variables.

The issues of data screening discussed in this article generally receive scant attention. Yet they concern strategic decisions that can have major implications for the ensuing results, as the criticism[11] of the Anturane study[12] has shown. They directly affect the validity and thus the ethics of research.

References

[1] "Student." The Lanarkshire milk experiment. *Biometrika* 1931;**23**: 398-406.

[2] Carleton RA, Sanders CA, Burack WR. Heparin administration after acute myocardial infarction. *N Engl J Med* 1960;**263**:1002-5.

[3] Peto R, Pike MC, Armitage P, *et al*. Design and analysis of randomized clinical trials requiring prolonged observation of each patient. I Introduction and design. *Br J Cancer* 1976;**34**:585-612.

[4] Clarke BF, Campbell IW. Long-term comparative trial of glibenclamide and chlorpropamide in diet-failed, maturity-onset diabetics. *Lancet* 1975;i:245-7.

[5] Healy MJR. The disciplining of medical data. *Br Med Bull* 1968;**24**:210-4.

[6] Armitage P. *Statistical methods in medical research.* Oxford: Blackwell, 1971:350-9.

[7] Flynn FV, Piper KAJ, Garcia-Webb P, McPherson K, Healy MJR. The frequency distributions of commonly determined blood constituents in healthy blood donors. *Clin Chim Acta* 1974;**52**:163-71.

[8] Carpenter RG, Emery JL. Final results of study of infants at risk of sudden death. *Nature* 1977;**268**:724-5.

[9] Meier P. The biggest health experiment ever: the 1954 field trial of the Salk poliomyelitis vaccine. In: Tanur JM, Mosteller F, Kruskal WH, *et al*, eds. *Statistics: a guide to the study of the biological and health sciences.* San Francisco: Holden-Day, 1977:88–100.

[10] Wilcox RG, Roland JM, Banks DC, Hampton JR, Mitchell JRA. Randomised trial comparing propranolol with atenolol in immediate treatment of suspected myocardial infarction. *Br Med J* 1980;**280**:885-8.

[11] Kolata GB. FDA says no to Anturane. *Science* 1980;**208**:1130-2.

[12] The Anturane Reinfarction Trial Research Group. Sulfinpyrazone in the prevention of sudden death after myocardial infarction. *N Engl J Med* 1980;**302**:250-6.

ANALYSING DATA

The incorrect analysis of data is probably the best known misuse of statistical methods, largely due to a series of reviews[1-3] that have shown how common such errors are in published papers. Nevertheless, these mistakes, which tend to be in the use of the simpler techniques, continue to proliferate. The mishandling of statistical analysis is as bad as the misuse of any laboratory technique. Both can lead to incorrect answers and conclusions and are thus unethical because they render research valueless.

I will look briefly at problems associated with simple significance tests and will consider in more depth some less well-appreciated difficulties associated with two other common techniques—correlation and regression. I will then look at two specific medical problems that often result in incorrect analyses.

Errors in common statistical analyses

Nowadays some types of statistical analyses are seen so often in medical publications that their use is taken for granted. Everyone knows them, but the evidence suggests that many people do not know how to use them properly, or when *not* to use them. For example, Gore *et al*[2] found at least one such error in about half of the papers containing statistical analyses that they reviewed.

t TESTS AND χ^2 TESTS

The *t* tests to compare two groups of measurements are used extremely widely, but often incorrectly.[2-4] The problems usually relate to the data not complying with the underlying statistical assumption that the two sets of data come from populations that are normal and have the same variance. Another serious error is to ignore the fact that the two sets of measurements relate to the same (or matched) individuals, in which case the paired *t* test is needed. These problems are fairly familiar and have been well illustrated by White[3] so I will not consider them further here.

Although generally posing fewer problems, χ^2 tests for comparing proportions also suffer some abuse, notably where there are too few observations. The sample size constraint also applies to the form of χ^2 test which simply entails comparing observed and expected frequencies. This method was used to compare observed numbers of deaths from five types of leukaemia (0, 1, 2, 4, 0) with their respective "expected" numbers (2, 1, 1, 3, 0),[5] but seven deaths is far too few for such an analysis to be valid.

CORRELATION

Perhaps one harmful side effect of the vast increase in availability of computing power is that the distinct statistical analyses of correlation and regression have become greatly confused. This is probably because of the close similarity between the mathematical calculations rather than for any logical reason, for it is relatively rare that one is truly interested in both analyses.

The correlation coefficient is a measure of the degree of linear (or "straight line") association between two continuous variables. If the relationship between the two variables is curved the correlation may be an artificially low measure of association. Alternatively, the correlation may be artificially high if a few observations are very different from the rest. For these reasons it is unwise to place any importance on the magnitude of the correlation without looking at a scatter plot of the data.

Misleading correlations can also be obtained if the data relate to different groups of subjects having different characteristics. Adam[6] looked at the relationship between body weight and the proportion of sleep that was rapid eye movement sleep in 16 adults, and found a rank correlation of 0·78. The original high correlation, however, was partly due to the men having higher values of both variables, for the correlations for men and women separately were 0·61 and 0·37 respectively. A further incorrect procedure is to use data comprising more than one observation per individual.

The main problem is that the test of significance of a correlation coefficient, which is a test of the null hypothesis of no association (zero correlation), is based on the assumption of joint normality of the two variables. This is characterised by the data points having a roughly elliptical shape in the scatter diagram. If this is not so the correlation will be misleading and the test of significance invalid. The distributional assumption may be overcome either by transformation of the data, or by the calculation of "rank" correlation, which makes no important assumptions.

In medical research correlations are greatly overused, perhaps because they are easy to calculate and are measured on a scale that is independent of the data. Correlation ought really to be considered to be mainly an investigative analysis, suggesting areas for further research; for forming hypotheses rather than for testing them.

REGRESSION

The rationale for regression analysis is very different. In regression we are interested in describing mathematically the dependence of one variable on one or more other variables. In the simple linear case we are calculating the equation of the "best" straight line relating to the so-called "dependent" variable (Y) to the "independent" (or explanatory) variable (X).* For example, we might be interested in the dependence of lung function on height or of blood pressure on age. The appropriateness of a linear relationship can again best be verified by means of a scatter plot.

The most important underlying assumption in regression is that the Y variable is normally distributed with the same variance for each value of X, and major departures from this condition can usually be detected by eye. There are no restrictions on X, so that it is perfectly valid, for example, to

*These terms simply denote which variable is considered to be dependent on the other.

choose a wide range of X values to get a better estimate of the regression line. This would, however, artificially inflate the correlation coefficient, although correlations are often calculated from such data.

Regression is used to estimate a dependence relationship. The resulting equation can be used to predict Y (say, lung function) from X (height) for an individual. The difference between an individual's actual and predicted lung functions can be used as a measure of lung function standardised for height.

Examples of improper practices are the use of the regression equation to predict the Y variable for values of the X variable outside the range of the original data set (called extrapolation); the fitting of a straight line where the data show curvature; the use of a Y on X regression equation to predict X from Y (except in certain circumstances); and the use of simple regression where there are heterogeneous subgroups (the correct technique being analysis of covariance). Unless there is a plot of the data most of these procedures may be undetectable in a published paper.

Method comparison studies

Some of the practical problems in analysing data, notably the choice of the correct analysis to match the relevant hypothesis, are well illustrated by the problems of method comparison studies.

In medical research it is quite common to carry out a study to compare two different methods of measuring something. This may be to compare measurements made with some new piece of equipment with the "true" measurements, but it is more often to compare two different measuring devices where neither can be said to give the truth. (A similar problem arises when comparing the same measurement on different occasions.)

The obvious first step in the analysis is to plot the values obtained by each method as a scatter diagram. To judge from publications, the apparently obvious second step is to calculate the correlation between the two measurements. This is, however, a completely misguided approach, stemming from the common failure to appreciate what information the correlation coefficient gives.

An example of the false reasoning that is very common in published work is given by a study[7] comparing two methods of assessing the gestational age of newborn babies; one was the much-used Dubowitz method based on neurological and physiological signs and the other the Robinson method, which is based on neurological signs only. The scatter diagram showed only moderate agreement. The correlation between the two methods, however, was 0·85, and the authors argued directly from this that the two methods agreed well and that it would be reasonable to use the simpler method.

To test an observed correlation coefficient for statistical significance is to test how likely the observed result would be under the "null hypothesis" that the two variables were not associated at all. This is patently ludicrous when the two variables are obviously associated by their very nature; we would be astonished to find that two methods of measurement were uncorrelated. In fact, it can be shown that in these circumstances the magnitude of the correlation largely reflects the spread of the measurements. As such, its use is completely erroneous in this context.

What we really want to know in these studies is how well the two measures agree. The simplest approach is to calculate the difference between two measurements for each subject. The mean of these differences will then be a measure of accuracy (or bias) and the standard deviation a measure of precision. Both bias and precision are necessary in order to assess agreement. The between-method differences may tend to increase as the measurements increase, in which case it may be necessary to transform the data before analysis. With more than two methods, or if repeat observations are made (which is desirable), the more general analysis of variance must be used.

Hunyor et al[8] did calculate the mean and standard deviation of paired differences when comparing various sphygmomanometric methods with intra-arterial blood pressures, but then based their statements about relative accuracy on the high correlations they found. They studied hypertensives only; had they studied some normotensives as well they would undoubtedly have observed higher correlations, but these would not have implied any better agreement between methods.

One last point about method comparison studies is that they are often carried out on such small numbers of subjects that the two methods will not be found significantly different unless there is an enormous difference between them. There is considerable potential here for incorrectly finding a new method acceptable, and for such methods to be recommended for widespread use without justification.

Reference ranges

Another area where simple statistical methods are often applied blindly is in the construction of reference (or normal) ranges against which to judge future observations. For example, some people believe that since a range is required, all that is needed is to obtain results from some "normal" subjects and quote the range of values. Apparent differences in reference ranges for the same index can often be attributed to one or more of them having been calculated incorrectly. Also, the sample size taken is often too small to get reliable answers. I have seen a reference range calculated from seven subjects, incorrectly at that, whereas at least 100 observations are needed to get a reliable range.

The usual calculation of a 95% reference range as the mean ±2 standard deviations is yet again based on the assumption that the data follow a Gaussian or normal distribution. Often this condition is not fulfilled and we see statements like "The mean ^{99m}Tc uptake in this group was 1·8% ± SD 1·1%, making the upper limit of normal (mean ± 2 SD) 4·0%."[9] The unstated lower limit is negative, however, which is nonsense. This type of calculation of a normal range on skew data results in considerably more than the nominal 5% of subjects being classified as "abnormal." The consequence of such a classification may be to perform further tests, so that there is a clear ethical aspect to the construction and interpretation of normal ranges. Even where the range is calculated sensibly there is a strong case for quoting the standard error of the limits, to emphasise the considerable uncertainty involved.

Whether or not the use of such ranges is sensible is beyond the scope of this article; the issues have been clearly discussed by Oldham[10] and Healy.[11]

Selecting which data to analyse

A rather more subtle problem that can occur in any study is the selection of which data to analyse. Errors may occur when analyses are carried out as a direct result of having seen the data. In a comparison of several groups of subjects it is not valid to select those groups with the highest and lowest values and apply the usual significance test to the means purely on that basis, because the null hypothesis of no difference is inappropriate when the largest difference is being examined. More generally, selection of comparisons to test because they "look interesting" will in the long run result in more than the nominal (say 5%) proportion of falsely positive results.

A second form of selection is to analyse only a subset of the subjects on the basis of their results. In a recent study 30 patients with idiopathic hypercalciuria were given a dietary supplement of unprocessed bran.[12] Only 22 patients "achieved a reduction in urinary calcium," and only these 22 patients were analysed. No data were provided on the other eight subjects, so we can not tell whether they really were a different group or just one end of a distribution of differing responses to the bran, which seems more likely. This procedure is completely unacceptable without justification—anyone can show significant results by analysing only those subjects with the greatest response.

The basic principle is to analyse according to the original hypothesis and experimental design. Other results that look interesting are pointers for further research.

Summary

It is of no value collecting good data if the analysis is inadequate or invalid. The results obtained may then be worthless, or at best they will fail to realise the true potential of the data. Either way, the value of the whole experiment is diminished to a point where the ethics of the investigation must be called into question.

References

[1] Schor S, Karten I. Statistical evaluation of medical journal manuscripts. *JAMA* 1966;**195**:1123-8.

[2] Gore SM, Jones IG, Rytter EC. Misuse of statistical methods: critical assessment of articles in *BMJ* from January to March 1976. *Br Med J* 1977;i:85-7.

[3] White SJ. Statistical errors in papers in the *British Journal of Psychiatry*. *Br J Psychiatry* 1979;**135**:336-42.

[4] Glantz SA. Biostatistics: how to detect, correct and prevent errors in the medical literature. *Circulation* 1980;**61**:1-7.

[5] Tabershaw IR, Lamm SH. Benzene and leukaemia. *Lancet* 1977;ii:867-8.

[6] Adam K. Bodyweight correlates with REM sleep. *Br Med J* 1977;i:813-4.

[7] Serfontein GL, Jaroszewicz AM. Estimation of gestational age at birth. *Arch Dis Child* 1978;**53**:509-11.

[8] Hunyor SN, Flynn JM, Cochineas C. Comparison of performance of various sphygmomanometers with intra-arterial blood pressure readings. *Br Med J* 1978;ii:159-62.

[9] Van 'T Hoff W, Pover GG, Eiser NM. Technetium-99^{m} in the diagnosis of thyrotoxicosis. *Br Med J* 1972;iv:203-6.

[10] Oldham PD. The uselessness of normal values. In: Arcangeli P, Cotes JE, Cournand A, eds. *Introduction to the definition of normal values for respiratory function in man*. Turin: Panminerva Medica, 1969:49-56.

[11] Healy MJR. Normal values from a statistical viewpoint. *Bullétin de l'Académie Royale de Médecine de Belgique* 1969;**9**:703-18.

[12] Shah PJR, Green NA, Williams G. Unprocessed bran and its effect on urinary calcium excretion in idiopathic hypercalciuria. *Br Med J* 1980;**281**:426.

PRESENTATION OF RESULTS

A very important aspect of statistical method is the clear numerical and graphical presentation of results. Although many statistical textbooks and courses discuss simple visual methods such as histograms, bar charts, pie charts, and so on, they are usually introduced as descriptive or investigative techniques. It is uncommon to find discussion of how best to present the results of statistical analyses. This is surprising, since the interpretation of the results, both by the researcher and by later readers of the paper, may be critically dependent on the methods used to present the results.

Little need be said here about the simple visual methods already mentioned—they are well covered by Huff.[1] The problems associated with graphs, however, are rather more important.

Graphical presentation

In 1976 a Government publication[2] gave examples of some past successes in preventive medicine. One of these examples concerned the introduction in the 1930s of mass immunisation against diphtheria. Figure 1(a) shows their presentation of childhood mortality from diphtheria from 1871 to 1971. This appears to show that the introduction of immunisation resulted in a rapid decline in mortality. In their figure, however, mortality is plotted on a logarithmic scale and shows proportional changes. When the data are plotted on a linear scale,[3] as in figure 1(b), the visual effect is quite different, as is the interpretation. From this figure we can see that over the period in question mortality from diphtheria had been dropping very quickly, and this specific preventive measure was adopted relatively late in the day. This is not to say that the introduction of immunisation was not effective, but that the degree of its effectiveness that one accepts depends considerably on which way the data are presented.

For experimental data it is unlikely to be appropriate to transform the scale of one or both axes unless it has been necessary to carry out the analysis on transformed data. For example, if analysis has been carried out on log data, it is probably better to show a scatter diagram with a log scale to demonstrate that the transformed data comply with the appropriate assumptions.

Scatter diagrams and regression

For simple data sets scatter diagrams are tremendously helpful. By showing all the data it is much easier for the reader to evaluate the analyses that were carried out. It is essential, however, that coincident points are indicated in some way. If there are different subgroups within the data set (different sexes perhaps) these may be indicated by means of different symbols. This will provide extra information at no expense, and will help to show the appropriateness (or otherwise) of analysing the data as one set, or for each subgroup separately.

Unfortunately, to many people scatter diagrams automatically suggest the calculation of correlations and the fitting of regression lines, even though one or both of these methods may be invalid or of no interest. One often sees scatter diagrams where a straight

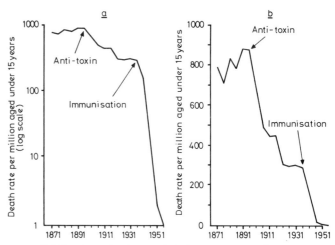

FIG 1—Childhood mortality from diphtheria (a) on a log scale[2] (b) on a linear scale.[3]

line has been drawn through the data but no reference is made to it, either in the figure or in the text. Perhaps the intention is to show that the data have been "properly analysed," but presentations like this demonstrate the reverse.

How should results of regression analyses be presented? This will depend partly on the context. For example, if the analysis shows that the relationship between two variables is too weak to be of practical value, then there may be little point in quoting the equation of the line of best fit. If the equation is given then the standard error of the slope (and of the intercept if this is of practical importance) and the number of observations are important information. One other quantity is necessary, however, before one can make full use of a regression equation. The equation can be used to estimate the variable Y for any new value of the variable X. Such an estimate is, however, of limited value without some measure of its uncertainty, for which it is additionally necessary to have the residual standard deviation.[4] This is a useful quantity in its own right, as it is a measure of the variability of the discrepancies (residuals) between the observations and the values predicted by the equation and is thus a measure of the "goodness of fit" of the regression line to the data. The residual standard deviation is rarely supplied in papers, so that it is impossible to know what uncertainty is attached to the use of the regression line for estimating Y from X.

Whatever information is presented, it is vital that it is unambiguous. The following equation may be meant to give much of the information but the meaning of the last term is unclear:

$$TBN(g) = (28 \cdot 8 * FFM(kg) + 288) \pm 8 \cdot 5\%.$$

The paper[5] from which this example comes also includes an example of a type of incorrect visual presentation of a regression equation—namely, the extension of the line well beyond the range of the data. This practice is extremely unreliable and potentially misleading, and can rarely be justified.

Variability

Despite its obvious importance and its almost universal presence in scientific papers, the presentation of variability in medical journals is a shambles. It is quite clear that some practices are now considered obligatory purely because they are widely used and accepted, not because they are particularly informative.

Much of the confusion may arise from imperfect appreciation of the difference between the standard deviation and the standard error. In simple terms the standard deviation is a measure of the variability of a set of observations, whereas the standard error is a measure of the precision of an estimate (mean, mean difference, regression slope, etc) in relation to its unknown true value. Despite this clear distinction in meaning, many people seem to have an innate preference for one or the other; some time ago I looked at all the issues of the *BMJ*, *Lancet*, and *New England Journal of Medicine* for October 1977 and found only three papers that used both, although 50 used either one or the other. Similar results were found in a much larger study.[6] It has been suggested that perhaps the standard error of the mean is more popular because it is always much smaller,[6 7] and this may well be so.

The standard deviation, which describes the variability of raw data, is often presented by attaching it to the corresponding mean using a $\pm$ sign: "The mean... was 30 mg (SD$\pm$4·6 mg)," or something similar. This presentation suggests that the standard deviation is $\pm$4·6 mg, but the standard deviation is always a positive number.[8] More importantly, it also suggests that the range from mean $-$SD to mean $+$SD (25·4 to 34·6 mg) is meaningful, but this is not so unless one is genuinely interested in the range encompassing about 68% of the observations. In general, the most useful range is probably the mean$\pm$2 SD, within which about 95% of the observations lie. This range is 20·8 to 39·2, which is twice as wide as that implied by "$\pm$4·6 mg." Such ranges apply only if the observations are approximately normally distributed. Otherwise, although the standard deviation can be calculated, it may not convey much information about the spread of the data. In such cases the median and two centiles (say the 10th and 90th or the 5th and 95th for larger samples) will provide better information.[9 10] The range of values may also be of interest, but it is highly dependent on the number of observations and is very sensitive to extreme or outlying observations. Alternatively, the omission of the $\pm$ sign leads to an unambiguous although much less informative presentation: "The mean was 30 mg (SD 4·6 mg)."

STANDARD ERRORS

Similar comments apply to the presentation of standard errors. Here the most often quoted range of $\pm$SE around an estimate is that within which we can be about 68% sure that the true value lies, whereas the 95% range is twice as wide. (For practical purposes these "confidence intervals" apply even when the data are not normally distributed). The presentation most usually used (mean$\pm$SE) is thus misleading in giving the impression of greater precision than has been achieved. Quoting the range mean$\pm$2 SE is much better, but this is rarely seen. Much confusion would be eliminated if the sign $\pm$ was used only when referring to a range.

ERROR BARS

Error bars are a popular way of displaying means and standard errors. They are usually a visual representation of the range mean$\pm$SE such as in figure 2. In this example the error bars for A and B do not overlap: does this tell us anything about the difference between the groups?

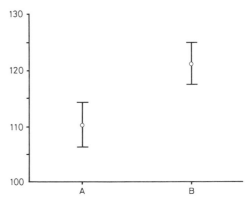

FIG 2—Mean ($\pm$SE) diastolic blood pressure from two sets of observations.

Suppose A and B represent two different types of sphygmomanometer, and we measure the diastolic pressure of 15 people using each machine. Figure 3(a) shows the results of such an experiment where the agreement is clearly good, but machine B tends to give slightly higher readings. Figure 3(b) shows some data where agreement is generally very poor. Yet both of these

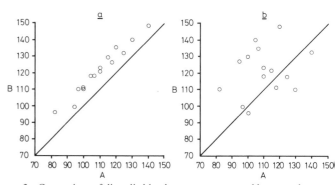

FIG 3—Comparison of diastolic blood pressures measured by two sphygmomanometers on 15 subjects (a) with good agreement but some bias, (b) with very poor agreement.

sets of data can be described exactly by the means and SEs in figure 2. This is because figure 2 tells us nothing about differences between machines for each subject. Error bars are thus useless in the case of paired observations.

Now suppose that we wish to compare the diastolic blood pressures of two distinct groups of people, say doctors (group A) and bus-drivers (group B). Figures 4(a) and 4(b) show two possible outcomes. In which case, if either, are the two groups significantly different? It is not easy to tell from the raw data shown that the groups are significantly different in figure 4(a) ($p < 0·05$) but not in figure 4(b) ($p > 0·1$). What would an "error-bar" plot show? Well, again both examples would yield figure 2, showing that the visual impression of non-overlapping bars does not by itself give any information about statistical significance. If the error bars do overlap, however, then the difference between the means is not statistically significant.[11]

For error bars to be useful they ought to convey useful information about either the precision of individual means or the differences between means. In their usual form they do neither, although my impression is that many people believe that they do both. The use of confidence intervals (mean$\pm$2 SE) instead of error bars does at least give useful information about individual means. Although it is sometimes possible to make the visual presentation give an indication of statistical significance, it is probably better to give confidence intervals and, if desired, report on the significance separately.

Numerical precision

One other aspect of presentation that deserves some comment is numerical precision. It is rarely necessary to quote results—

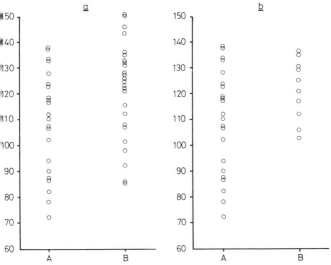

FIG 4 (a) and (b)—Comparisons of diastolic blood pressure in two different groups of subjects.

means, standard deviations, and so on—to more than three significant figures (that is, excluding leading or trailing zeros). For tabular presentation it may be a positive advantage to reduce the precision of each entry to make any patterns or trends more obvious.[12]

Spurious precision should also be avoided. Examples are the quoting of t or χ^2 values to four decimal places, and a regression slope with seven significant figures (12·97642). My favourite is the summary[13] of a test of significance as $p < 10^{-54}$, although I must concede that there is only one significant figure here!

Some suggestions

More thought should be given to numerical and visual presentation, rather than automatically following precedent. Some ways of supplying more information without using more space are:

(1) In a plot information about the spread of data (by ± 2 SD ranges or centiles) can be given as well as means and confidence intervals.

(2) A figure and a table may be combined by using the X axis labels as table column headings. For example, in fig 2 I could have given the mean, SD, range, and sample size for the two groups under the figure using little extra space.

(3) When scatter plots have the same variable on each axis as in figure 3(a) and 3(b), a small histogram of the within-person differences can be added in an otherwise empty corner.

Summary

Whatever results are presented it is vital that the methods are identified. In one survey of over 1000 papers[14] as many as 20% of the procedures were unidentified, and in another it was not clear whether the SD or SE was given in 11% of 608 papers.[6] It is impossible to appraise a paper in the presence of such ambiguities.

Visual display is a particularly effective way of presenting results. Given alternatives, however, many people might opt for the method of display that fits in better with their beliefs. If decisions are taken as a result of such presentations then there is scope for manipulating events by choice of presentation. This practice is well recognised in the way statistics are sometimes presented in the mass media and advertisements; we should not rule out this phenomenon in the medical world.

References

[1] Huff D. *How to lie with statistics*. Harmondsworth: Penguin, 1973.
[2] Department of Health and Social Security. *Prevention and health: everybody's business*. London: HMSO, 1976.
[3] Radical Statistics Health Group. *Whose priorities?* London: Radical Statistics, 1976.
[4] Armitage P. *Statistics in medical research*. Oxford: Blackwell, 1971:150-6.
[5] Hill GL, Bradley JA, Collins JP, McCarthy I, Oxby CB, Burkinshaw L. Fat-free body mass from skinfold thickness: a close relationship with total body nitrogen. *Br J Nutr* 1978;**39**:403-5.
[6] Bunce H, Hokanson JA, Weiss GB. Avoiding ambiguity when reporting variability in biomedical data. *Am J Med* 1980;**69**:8-9.
[7] Glantz SA. Biostatistics: how to detect, correct and prevent errors in the medical literature. *Circulation* 1980;**61**:1-7.
[8] Gardner MJ. Understanding and presenting variation. *Lancet* 1975;i:230-1.
[9] Mainland D. SI units and acidity. *Br Med J* 1977;ii:1219-20.
[10] Feinstein AR. Clinical biostatistics. XXXVII Demeaned errors, confidence games, nonplussed minuses, inefficient coefficients, and other statistical disruptions of scientific communication. *Clin Pharmacol Ther* 1976;**20**:617-31.
[11] Browne RH. On visual assessment of the significance of a mean difference. *Biometrics* 1979;**35**:657-65.
[12] Ehrenberg ASC. Rudiments of numeracy. *Journal of the Royal Statistical Society* Series A 1977;**140**:277-97.
[13] Vaughan Williams EM, Tasgal J, Raine AEG. Morphometric changes in rabbit ventricular myocardium produced by long-term beta-adrenoceptor blockade. *Lancet* 1977;ii:850-2.
[14] Feinstein AR. Clinical biostatistics. XXV A survey of the statistical procedures in general medical journals. *Clin Pharmacol Ther* 1974;**15**:97-107.

INTERPRETING RESULTS

"... it is a function of statistical method to emphasise that precise conclusions cannot be drawn from inadequate data."

E S PEARSON AND H O HARTLEY[1]

The problems of interpretation have already appeared several times in the preceding pages. Obviously the sorts of error already discussed, most likely in design or analysis, may lead to incorrect results and thus erroneous conclusions. But some errors are specific to the interpretation of results, and these I will consider now. Most emphasis will be given to tests of significance, since these quite clearly cause great difficulty.

Significance tests

Before tackling some of the trickier issues it is worth making the general point that the sensible interpretation of statistical analysis cannot be independent of the knowledge of what the data are (and how they were obtained).

Table I, for example, shows the results of the comparison of two groups of subjects given different treatments with the outcome for each subject recorded as positive or negative, where both outcomes would be expected to be equally likely.

TABLE I—*Comparison of outcomes for two treatment groups*

		Outcome +	Outcome −	Total
Treatment	1	4	4	8
	2	8	24	32
Total		12	28	40

Obviously the group 1 results were as expected, whereas for group 2 a χ^2 test shows a significant excess of negative outcomes, but in the absence of further information we are unable to interpret these results. Knowing that the subjects were all pregnant and the outcomes were male and female babies is likely to aid interpretation and increase interest, but the further knowledge that the subjects were all cows will probably lessen interest again, unless you are a farmer. Yet you may be curious to know what the "treatments" were—perhaps there is some relevance for people. Well, all the cows were artificially inseminated; those in group 1 were facing north at the time and those in group 2 were facing south.[2]

Given all the information, most people would probably dismiss this as a chance finding, rather than accept it as evidence of an association between the direction the cows were facing and the sex of their calves. This is quite reasonable behaviour if we consider the meaning of statistical significance.

INTERPRETING SIGNIFICANT RESULTS

Like several statistical terms, "significant" is perhaps an ill-chosen one. It should be realised that the level of significance is just an indication of the degree of plausibility of the "null

hypothesis," which in the above example was that the outcomes of the two groups were really the same. If the null hypothesis is deemed too implausible we reject it and accept the "alternative hypothesis" that the treatments differ in their effect.

It is ridiculous to lay down rigid rules for something so subjective, especially as interpretation will be greatly influenced by other evidence—few studies are carried out in isolation. As Box *et al*[3] have said: "If the alternative hypothesis were plausible a priori, the experimenter would feel much more confident of a result significant at the 0·05 level than if it seemed to contradict all previous experience." Indeed, in the long run one in 20 comparisons of equally effective treatments will be significant at the 5% level (by definition), so to accept all significant results as real[4] is extremely unwise, as the above data illustrate.

Conventional significance levels (5%, 1%, 0·1%) are useful, but only as guides to interpretation, not as strict rules. To describe a result of p=0·05 as "probably significant"[5] implies that the interpretation depends on which side of 0·05 p really is. On the contrary, values of p of, say, 0·06 and 0·04 should not lead to opposite conclusions, but to closely similar ones.

One prevalent misconception relates to the precise meaning of p, the significance level; p is the probability of obtaining a result at least as unlikely as the observed one, if the null hypothesis of no effect is true. The last part of this definition is essential; to omit it leads to the common error of believing that p is also the probability so that we make a mistake by accepting the significant result as a real finding. This is just not so, and it is sad to see this view in a paper trying to explain the meaning of significance.[6] All we can say is that p is the probability of such a result arising if the null hypothesis is true. We obviously do not actually know whether the null hypothesis *is* true, so the probability of rejecting it in error is also unknown, although this clearly reduces as p gets smaller.

INTERPRETING NON-SIGNIFICANT RESULTS

Every significance test measures the credibility of a null hypothesis—for example, that two treatments are equally effective. A non-significant result just means that the results were not strong enough to reject the null hypothesis; "not significant" does not imply either "not important" or "non-existent." To consider all non-significant results as indicating no effect of importance is clearly wrong. Conversely, to believe that an observed difference is a real one with an insufficient degree of certainty is to run a large risk of chasing shadows. Thus when reporting "negative" results, it is especially important to give a confidence interval around the observed effect[7 8]—for example, around the difference between two means.

In "How large a sample?" (page 6) I discussed at length the idea of the power of a significance test. It is appropriate to return to the topic of power here. Studies with low power (as a result of inadequate sample size) will often yield results showing effects which, if real, would be of clinical importance, but which are not statistically significant. In general it is safest to consider such non-significant results as being inconclusive (or "not proven"), preferably backed up with a recommendation that further data be collected. When this is not feasible and there are ethical implications, as in the following example, the problem of interpretation is particularly great.

Carpenter and Emery[9] investigated the possible effect on the incidence of sudden unexpected infant death of an increase in the number of visits by the health visitor to high-risk babies. They found fewer unexplained deaths in the "treatment" group (five out of 837) than in the control group (nine out of 922), but the difference is not nearly statistically significant ($p > 0.5$). From a statistical point of view, the results are inconclusive. Because such deaths are rare, the power of the study was very low; it would have needed a much larger sample to get a clear answer.[10] The authors asked: "Can we reasonably withhold increased surveillance from all high-risk infants?"[11] More dispassionately we might ask whether the evidence is really strong enough to justify a change in policy that would presumably necessitate withdrawing health visitors from other activities.

MULTIPLE TESTS OF SIGNIFICANCE

A further difficulty arises when several tests of significance are carried out on one set of data. This may, for example, take the form of looking to see which pairs of a number of groups are significantly different from each other, or which of a number of different factors are related to a variable of interest. Unfortunately, the greater the number of tests carried out, the higher the overall risk of a "false-positive" result. As Meier has pointed out,[12] it is not reasonable to restrict the number of aspects of the data that are investigated purely to relieve the statistician's problems of interpretation. He suggested a good compromise, which is to treat a small number of tests as being of primary importance, "and to regard other findings as tentative, subject to confirmation in future experiments." The level of significance will have some bearing here, since we will be more ready to accept a highly significant finding (say, $p < 0.001$) even in the context of numerous tests.

Association and causation

It is widely believed that "you can prove *anything* with statistics," but it is much more realistic to say that you can establish *nothing* by statistics alone. This is especially true when considering the interpretation of observed associations between two variables. It is easy and often tempting to assume that the underlying relationship is a causal one, even in the absence of any supporting evidence, but many associations are not causal. In particular, misleading associations appear when each of the variables is correlated with a third "hidden" variable. A simple example of this phenomenon is when two variables that change with time display an association in the complete absence of any causal relationship—for example, the divorce rate and the price of petrol.

The deduction of a causal relationship from an observed association can rarely be justified from the data alone. Support is needed from prior knowledge, including other experimental or observational data. Sometimes, however, such information is not obtainable, and the causal hypothesis can be supported only by allowing for the most likely hidden variables. There are several examples of epidemiological studies producing associations that are not unanimously believed to be causal, such as that between water hardness and cardiovascular mortality. A few people do not even accept that the association between smoking and lung cancer is causal despite the great volume of collateral evidence.

A recent paper[13] concerning the failure to show a relationship between diet and serum cholesterol concentration gave a salutary reminder that variables may falsely appear to be unrelated. Although a strong relationship between dietary cholesterol and serum cholesterol has been shown in closely controlled dietary studies, the authors showed that a straightforward population study would be likely to miss such an association because of several sources of variability in both variables.

Another difficulty that can beset the interpretation of observed associations is where two possibly causal factors are inseparable. A simple example is where two alternative methods of measurement are compared with only one experimenter using each method.[14] Any observed differences may be due either to differences between the methods or between the experimenters, or both. The two effects are *confounded*. A much more complex version of the same problem arises when trying to explain different mortality rates for the same disease in different countries.

Prediction

The use of observed relationships to make predictions about individuals is another area with many pitfalls. Just as it is dangerous to generalise from the particular, we must be very careful about particularising from the general.

For continuous variables, relationships are usually described by regression equations. It must be remembered that such fitted equations are approximate, both because they are calculated from a sample of data, and also because the imposition of an exact relationship (straight-line or curved) may be more convenient than realistic. The degree of scatter of the observations around the fitted line indicates the closeness of the relationship between the variables, and thus the uncertainty associated with predicting one from the other for specific cases. For example, a regression of height on weight for adult men would show a clear positive relationship with a large amount of scatter.

Regression equations should be used for prediction only within their limitations, so the regression line described above would be inappropriate for either boys or women. Such extrapolation is completely invalid. Also the prediction of height would be more certain for someone of average weight than for a very light or very heavy man, and this is borne out by the correct 95% confidence intervals for prediction which become wider further from the mean. It is very common to see a single figure quoted for the precision of any possible estimate; this is quite wrong.

Prediction also poses problems where the data are categorical. Table II shows the relationship between two diagnostic tests and the presence or absence of two diseases. Data such as these are usually described by the sensitivity and specificity, confusing terms for the proportions of correctly diagnosed positives and negatives. In both cases the sensitivity and specificity are high at 0.9 (maximum 1.0). These do not, however, measure the value of such tests for predictive purposes; in fact they become more misleading the lower the prevalence of the disease. The best approach is to consider what proportions of the diagnosed positives and negatives were true positives and negatives respectively. In table IIa, where the prevalence is 50%, these figures are also both 0.9, indicating high predictive ability. In table IIb, the prevalence is 2%. Although virtually all of those with a negative test were truly negative (4410/4420), only 16% (90/580) of those diagnosed as positive were true positives. So the value of the test is low, even though 90% of the true positives give positive results. The usefulness of such a test depends on the cost of a false-positive finding. This is the problem when deciding whether or not screening for rare conditions (such as breast cancer) is worth while. For such purposes, the sensitivity is of no use at all—a high sensitivity is a necessary but not sufficient condition for a good predictive test.

Exactly the same considerations apply to the interpretation of a value exceeding a reference (or normal) range as automatically indicating abnormality without consideration of the prevalence of abnormality. Indeed, this is equivalent to looking at only the

TABLE II—*Relation between diagnostic test and disease state with prevalence of disease (a) 50% and (b) 2%*

(a)		Test +	Test −		(b)		Test +	Test −	
Disease	+	180	20	200	Disease	+	90	10	100
	−	20	180	200		−	490	4410	4900
		200	200	400			580	4420	5000

top row in table IIb. Such a procedure can lead to ludicrous interpretations of data—for example, that it is safer to drive very fast as few accidents are caused by cars travelling at more than 100 miles an hour.

Conclusions

The enormous amount of published research makes it inevitable that papers will often be judged, in the first instance at least, by the authors' own conclusions or summary. It is thus vitally important that these contain valid interpretations of the results of the study, since the publication of misleading conclusions may both nullify the research in question and falsely influence medical practice and further research.

References

[1] Pearson ES, Hartley HO. *Biometrika tables for statisticians.* Vol 1. 3rd ed. Cambridge: University Press, 1970: 83.

[2] Wood PDP. On the importance of correct orientation to sex in cattle. *Statistician* 1977;**26**:304-6.

[3] Box GEP, Hunter WG, Hunter JS. *Statistics for experimenters.* New York: Wiley, 1978:109.

[4] Dudley H. When is significant not significant? *Br Med J* 1977;ii:47.

[5] Newton J, Illingworth R, Elias J, McEwan J. Continuous intrauterine copper contraception for three years: comparison of replacement at two years with continuation of use. *Br Med J* 1977;i:197-9.

[6] Glantz SA. Biostatistics: how to detect, correct and prevent errors in the medical literature. *Circulation* 1980;**61**:1-7.

[7] Rose G. Beta-blockers in immediate treatment of myocardial infarction. *Br Med J* 1980;**280**:1088.

[8] Chalmers TC, Matta RJ, Smith H, Kunzler A-M. Evidence favoring the use of anticoagulants in the hospital phase of acute myocardial infarction. *N Engl J Med* 1977;**297**:1091-6.

[9] Carpenter RG, Emery JL. Final results of study of infants at risk of sudden death. *Nature* 1977;**268**:724-5.

[10] Bland JM. Assessment of risk of sudden death in infants. *Nature* 1978;**273**:74.

[11] Carpenter RG, Emery JL. Reply to J M Bland. *Nature* 1978;**273**:74-5.

[12] Meier P. Statistics and medical experimentation. *Biometrics* 1975;**31**:511-29.

[13] Jacobs DR, Anderson JT, Blackburn H. Diet and serum cholesterol: do zero correlations negate the relationship? *Am J Epidemiol* 1979;**110**:77-87.

[14] Serfontein GL, Jaroszewicz AM. Estimation of gestational age at birth. *Arch Dis Child* 1978;**53**:509-11.

IMPROVING THE QUALITY OF STATISTICS IN MEDICAL JOURNALS

Publication of a paper implies that the work is both sound and worth while. As I pointed out in my first article, it bestows both respectability and credibility on the work—a "seal of approval." Once a paper has been published the results may influence both medical practice and further research by other scientists, and if the subject is of general interest the "mass media" may report the findings.

The ultimate responsibility for the general standard of published research rests with the medical journals. Perhaps unwillingly, the journals have the role of guardians of quality. This is particularly important with regard to statistical methods, which the majority of readers of medical papers are not able to judge for themselves and so must take on trust. The system of appraisal by independent referees is not ideal, but it is probably the most practical method of quality control. Referees are usually selected, however, for their expertise in the relevant medical topic; their ability to assess the statistical aspects is left somewhat to chance. The result is that the statistical methods used in many research papers do not receive adequate scrutiny, with the consequences described in the previous articles.

The poor quality of statistics in published papers has been a cause of concern for many years, and is not confined to medical research. In 1964 Yates and Healy[1] wrote: "It is depressing to find how much good biological work is in danger of being wasted through incompetent and misleading analysis of numerical results." Concern should be particularly great in the medical field because of the ethical implications, but the medical journals have generally been slow to appreciate that the statistical aspects can be fundamental to the validity of research.

Statistics in medical papers

Probably as a reflection of widespread unease, there have been several reviews of the quality of statistics in published papers over the past 15 years.[2-6] These views are not strictly comparable because they looked at different statistical aspects in different journals at different times. Nevertheless, they all found many statistical errors or important errors of omission—in 72%, 49%, 52%, 45%, and 44% of papers studied, respectively. Further, a review of papers in five general medical journals found that 20% of the statistical procedures used were unidentified.[7]

It is impossible to assess the seriousness of many of the errors found. For example, an invalid analysis *may* give the same answer as an appropriate one, omission of information about randomisation does not necessarily mean that subjects were not allocated to treatments at random, and so on. It is, though, a measure of the disturbingly high prevalence of bad statistics that the reviewers of 62 papers in the *BMJ*[4] thought that it was "some comfort that only five papers drew a false conclusion."

Reviews of statistical procedures have sometimes been accompanied by editorials[8 9] reinforcing the suggestions made in most of the papers that the standards of teaching should be improved and that there should be greater participation by statisticians in medical research. Such articles, however, stop short of the obvious suggestion that many of the papers should not have been published, at least as they stood, since any errors

detected after publication could equally well have been detected at the refereeing stage.

Not all journals are equally culpable. The number of journals that use statisticians as referees, and sometimes also as members of editorial boards, has gradually increased, and several journals have publicly recognised the need to improve their statistical reviewing.[10-12] As Rennie[10] says: "Our goal is the publication of data that are correctly observed and properly analysed." Such sentiments should be endorsed by all medical journals.

Raising statistical standards

Later I shall examine in some detail what the journals can do to improve standards. It is, however, important to realise that there are other aspects to the problem, which can broadly be summarised by the question: "Why is the standard of statistics so low in papers *submitted* for publication?"

TEACHING OF STATISTICS

The recent widespread move to include statistics in the syllabus for medical students and other science undergraduates is a welcome development. Such teaching is likely to be most beneficial when it gets away from a rigid method-orientated approach and concentrates more on general concepts. For medical students it may be more successful when not taught as an isolated subject, but closely related to another course such as epidemiology.[13]

Statistics is not an easy subject, however. A short introductory course is not sufficient to equip qualified doctors or scientists to carry out their own statistical analyses adequately, both because of the necessarily limited scope of such courses and also because several years may elapse before they need to use the knowledge. Thus although there is room for improvement in undergraduate teaching, it is unlikely to have much effect on the quality of statistics in medical research.

Of greater value in this respect would be postgraduate courses in statistics for those who had previously had an introductory course, and aimed particularly at those intending to do research. Such courses should try to give a greater understanding of statistical concepts: to help researchers to understand properly the simpler statistical methods (including when not to use them), to appreciate the principles of more advanced methods, and to know when to seek expert help. If such courses exist they are rare.

Similar comments apply to textbooks, where there is a wide gap between the elementary[14] and the comprehensive.[15] Simple textbooks are usually much too strongly method-orientated to give a good grasp of the underlying principles behind much of statistics.

INVOLVEMENT OF STATISTICIANS

In general, the larger a project the more likely it is that a statistician will be directly concerned. Yet a survey[16] of 211 cancer treatment studies in progress in 1978 showed that in only 47% was a statistician fully concerned (in design, data collection, and analysis). There was some involvement in a further 44%, but in 9% there was none. Unfortunately, not all medical researchers have direct access to a statistician, but large collaborative studies usually need considerable statistical advice,[17] preferably with a statistician as an active participant. Even for small studies statistical advice before the research begins may be very valuable, especially in helping to match the design to the objectives of the study, and also to give the statistician a greater understanding of the research. Yet, despite common pleas for early involvement, most consultancy concerns the analysis of data that have already been collected. A bigger problem, though, is that many projects are carried out without the benefit of any statistical advice at all. Increased involvement of statisticians in medical research would clearly improve the overall standard of statistics, but this requires greater availability of medical statisticians than at present.

Successful consultancy relies on the ability of both researcher and statistician to understand each other's language, which is not always easy. Sprent[18] has suggested that "Interdisciplinary communication is probably the most pressing problem in the pursuit of knowledge." The difficulties from the statistician's viewpoint have been discussed so often that a 1977 bibliography[19] gave nearly 40 references. One aspect not often mentioned is that statisticians receive little or no preparation for consultancy work, either with respect to the sort of practical statistical problems that arise, or the role of consultant. This is a definite shortcoming in the education of statisticians, especially important because of their influence on the conduct of medical research.

ETHICAL COMMITTEES

Ethical committees have the opportunity to review many protocols for intended research on human subjects, and have the important sanction of withholding their approval. In view of the ease with which research can be rendered unethical by statistical mismanagement (as discussed in previous articles) it should be an automatic part of the review by ethical committees to look formally at the experimental design, and preferably also at the intended form of analysis. May[20] has written: "A poorly designed or poorly conceived experiment is unethical by definition and should not be permitted. Further it is the responsibility of the review committee to ensure that the conception and design meet the accepted canons of scientific method because we are dealing with experimentation which may not be for the individual subject's direct benefit." We can share his surprise that statisticians are not universally represented on ethical committees.

WHY PUBLISH?

One reason for the relentless production of low quality papers (not only with respect to the statistics) is the pressure on many individuals to publish as much as possible, with quantity being much more important than quality. At present it is known that other papers with poor statistics are being published, so a scientist may well think that there is no incentive (or need) to do better. But if journals were more careful about what they published we might advance to a state where fewer papers of a higher standard were produced. This might also help to stem the counter-productive flow of new journals.

Role of the medical journals

There is general agreement among the medical journals in their attitude towards publishing the results of unethical research. Such research may have yielded valuable findings, but, as one editor wrote[21]: "publication in a reputable journal automatically implies that the editor and his reviewers condone the experimentation." In effect, papers describing unethical research are treated as "inadmissible evidence." For papers that may be deemed unethical because of their incorrect use of statistical methods, however, the attitudes of the journals vary enormously. Surely the same sort of argument as above should be extended, with publication similarly implying editorial approval of the data analysis and interpretation of results. It is illogical to refuse (quite rightly) to publish possibly useful findings of unethical research and yet be prepared to publish papers in which the results are invalidated by incorrect use of statistical methods.

One of the more obvious dangers of publishing questionable papers is that the conclusions may be quoted uncritically in the national press (since journalists are not usually qualified to criticise). Any ensuing critical letters will not receive similar publicity.

STATISTICAL REVIEW OF PAPERS

Since the reviews of published papers[2-6] have found errors in about half of the papers examined, it is obvious that statistical review *before* publication ought to be highly effective. In 1964 the *Journal of the American Medical Association* raised the proportion of published papers considered statistically acceptable from one-third to three-quarters when it introduced a comprehensive statistical reviewing procedure.[22]

Some of the following suggestions about ways in which journals can raise the quality of statistics in published papers have been made before,[6 11 22] most notably in two recent papers.[23 24] The most important recommendations are:

Statisticians should help referee

Journals should recruit statistically experienced people as referees, preferably with representation on editorial boards. Statistical review should be a formal procedure and not based on a casual inquiry to the nearest available statistician to "check that everything is all right." This is particularly important for specialist journals, where some depth of knowledge of the subject is often necessary.

All papers using any statistical procedure should be refereed by a statistician

Any paper in which inferences are drawn from the data presented should be seen by a statistician, whatever the level of statistical content. Indeed, the papers that cause the most trouble are usually those using only simple statistical methods ". . . where formal statistical review had seemed unwarranted,"[10] rather than those with more complicated analyses. Short reports should not be exempt but should get higher priority. To reduce the work load the statistical assessment could be carried out only when a paper is likely to prove otherwise acceptable.

Revised papers should be returned to the same referee for reappraisal

A statistical refereeing system cannot work well without this condition. Failure to do this was the main reason why only 75% of published papers were completely acceptable even after the introduction of such a scheme.[22]

Journals using a statistical refereeing system should state clearly what their policy is

This may help to discourage the submission of poor papers, and it would be valuable information for readers to know whether or not a journal uses such a system.

There should be statistical guidelines for contributors

All journals have instructions for contributors; very few mention statistics, and these rarely say much. It would obviously be undesirable for each journal to have different guidelines, but some agreement on this could be achieved in the same way as it has been on formats for references, perhaps in collaboration with the statistical societies. Some suggestions are given below.

All research papers should include a separate section on statistical methods

This should include information on relevant aspects of design, data collection, and analysis. Particularly important (if relevant) are the treatment allocation policy, response rate (and how non-responders were dealt with), and clear descriptions of analyses. Unusual methods of analysis should be given a specific reference (not a whole textbook!) with the reason for their use. This is a very important section of a paper, and should not be shortened at the expense of essential information.

Journals should give priority to well-executed and well-documented studies

Editorial boards should carefully consider the quality of study design, performance, analysis, and presentation of results when evaluating manuscripts. Standards should not be relaxed just because a paper is topical or interesting. Also, journals should not reject statistically valid papers purely because the findings were negative. (Obviously, this does not extend to those studies, discussed in "How large a sample?" (page 6), that are too small to detect important differences.) As Bradford Hill said 25 years ago: "A negative result may be dull but often it is no less important than the positive; and in view of that importance it must, surely, be established by adequate publication of the evidence."[25]
Less important but still desirable additional features are:

Authors should be encouraged to supply additional information (especially on methodology) to help the referees but not for publication

One of the problems when assessing papers is lack of information necessary for proper statistical assessment; this is the main reason for the sixth recommendation above. The extra information could be a more detailed account of the design, a fuller description of the methods used and the results, and copies of other related papers.

Authors should be encouraged to include the raw data in their papers

Obviously this is only practicable for small studies, but could be eased by using "miniprint" tables.

Journals should employ editorial staff with some understanding of statistics

This is perhaps less important if a comprehensive statistical refereeing system is adopted but is still highly desirable, especially in the event of disagreement between authors and referees.
For all journals to implement a comprehensive statistical refereeing system might well require many more medical statisticians than are currently available. It is much more likely, however, that there will be a continued steady increase in the use of statistical referees by journals, which should not cause major problems. Even the appointment by a journal of a single statistician can be enormously successful in raising the quality of statistics in published papers.

GUIDELINES FOR STATISTICAL REFEREES

Apart from checking on the validity of the statistical methods used, referees should ensure that there is adequate explanation and justification of what was done. It is also particularly important that the conclusions are reasonable, and that the summary is a fair reflection of the content.
The referee's report should be able to be understood by the authors, who may have only minimal statistical training.

GUIDELINES FOR CONTRIBUTORS

What sort of statistical guidelines should journals provide? Clearly these should not include advice on how to carry out research, although they might include discussion of the merits of different types of design. Such guidelines would not be a set of rules, but rather advice. The main emphasis should be on how best to describe clearly what procedures were used and what inferences were drawn.
Comprehensive guidelines would be of great benefit; these could perhaps be produced by a working party including representatives of medical journals and statistical societies. The following general suggestions relate to some of the more important aspects; they cannot be taken as comprehensive.
Design—This should be described clearly with, if relevant, information on treatment allocation, sample selection, if and how randomisation was used, whether or not the study was "blind" in any way, how sample size was determined (power), etc.
Data collection—Surveys should have response rates specified, and the representativeness of the sample and the possible effects of non-response should be discussed.
Analysis—The use of unusual forms of analysis should be justified, preferably with a reference, but all analyses should be very clearly described. It may be necessary to demonstrate the validity of the assumptions for some analyses (t tests, regression, etc).
Presentation of results—The results presented should be those most relevant to the question asked. Thus analysis of paired data should be accompanied by information—for instance, mean and standard deviation—about the within-person differences. Significance levels should not be given in place of quantitative results.
Interpretation of results—Special care should be taken to distinguish between statistical significance and clinical significance. Confidence intervals may greatly aid interpretation, especially where results are not statistically significant.

CONCLUSIONS

Reviews of published papers[2-6] have all found unacceptably high proportions of papers with statistical errors. Some journals may feel that their policy of publishing letters criticising individual papers is an adequate safeguard. To take this attitude is to fail to appreciate the responsibility of the journals, both for ethical and scientific reasons, to avoid publishing sub-standard papers. In any case letters to journals usually produce a reply from the authors repeating their incorrect claims. Further, most papers are never read by anyone with the statistical knowledge to detect the flaws. If the credibility of published research is to be raised it is essential that more journals introduce comprehensive statistical review procedures.

Summary

In this series I have concentrated very much on one aspect of research. This is not meant to imply that statistics is of overriding importance, but rather that it is an area where much improvement is both highly desirable and possible.
By emphasising the ethical implications of carrying out research and publishing papers with incorrect statistics, I have argued that this is not just a matter for the individual researcher. There needs to be a wider appreciation of the importance of correct statistical thinking, and a great improvement in the standard of published research so that the sorts of errors discussed become very much the exception rather than commonplace. In the long term improved teaching and the greater

involvement of statisticians will help; in the short term it is essential to have higher standards for published papers.

References

[1] Yates F, Healy MJR. How should we reform the teaching of statistics? *Journal of the Royal Statistical Society A* 1964;**127**:199-210.

[2] Schor S, Karten I. Statistical evaluation of medical journal manuscripts. *JAMA* 1966;**195**:1123-8.

[3] Lionel NDW, Herxheimer A. Assessing reports of therapeutic trials. *Br Med J* 1970;iii:637-40.

[4] Gore SM, Jones IG, Rytter EC. Misuse of statistical methods: critical assessment of articles in *BMJ* from January to March 1976. *Br Med J* 1977;i:85-7.

[5] White SJ. Statistical errors in papers in the *British Journal of Psychiatry*. *Br J Psychiatry* 1979;**135**:336-42.

[6] Glantz SA. Biostatistics: how to detect, correct, and prevent errors in the medical literature. *Circulation* 1980;**61**:1-7.

[7] Feinstein AR. Clinical biostatistics. XXV A survey of the statistical procedures in general medical journals. *Clin Pharmacol Ther* 1974;**15**:97-107.

[8] Anonymous. A pillar of medicine. *JAMA* 1966;**195**:1145.

[9] Anonymous. Statistical errors. *Br Med J* 1977;i:66.

[10] Rennie D. Vive la différence (p < 0·05). *N Engl J Med* 1978;**299**:828-9.

[11] Shuster JJ, Binion J, Moxley J, *et al.* Statistical review process. Recommended procedures for biomedical research articles. *JAMA* 1976;**235**:534-5.

[12] Rosen MR, Hoffman BF. Statistics, biomedical scientists, and *Circulation Research*. *Circ Res* 1978;**42**:739.

[13] Clarke M, Clayton DG, Donaldson LJ. Teaching epidemiology and statistics to medical students—the Leicester experience. *Int J Epidemiol* 1980;**9**:179-85.

[14] Swinscow TDV. *Statistics at square one*. London: BMA, 1976.

[15] Armitage P. *Statistical methods in medical research*. Oxford: Blackwell, 1971.

[16] Tate HC, Rawlinson JB, Freedman LS. Randomised comparative studies in the treatment of cancer in the United Kingdom: room for improvement? *Lancet* 1979;ii:623-5.

[17] Breslow N. Perspectives on the statistician's role in cooperative clinical research. *Cancer* 1978;**41**:326-32.

[18] Sprent P. Some problems of statistical consultancy (with discussion). *Journal of the Royal Statistical Society A* 1970;**133**:139-64.

[19] Woodward WA, Schucany WR. Bibliography for statistical consulting. *Biometrics* 1977;**33**:564-5.

[20] May WW. The composition and function of ethical committees. *J Med Ethics* 1975;**1**:23-9.

[21] Woodford FP. Ethical experimentation and the editor. *N Engl J Med* 1972;**286**:892.

[22] Schor S. Statistical reviewing program for medical manuscripts. *American Statistician* 1967;**21**:28-31.

[23] O'Fallon JR, Dubey SD, Salsburg DS, Edmonson JH, Soffer A, Colton T. Should there be statistical guidelines for medical research papers? *Biometrics* 1978;**34**:687-95.

[24] Mosteller F, Gilbert JP, McPeek B. Reporting standards and research strategies for controlled trials. Agenda for the editor. *Controlled Clinical Trials* 1980;**1**:37-58.

[25] Hill AB. Contribution to the discussion of a paper by D J Finney. *Journal of the Royal Statistical Society A* 1956;**119**:19-20.

I am especially grateful to Martin Bland, Ted Coles, Stewart Mann, Charles Rossiter, and Patrick Royston for their perceptive criticism of earlier drafts. I must also thank Nicola Wilson Smith for the large amount of typing she has done.

STATISTICS IN QUESTION

SHEILA M GORE MA PHD

Medical statistician, MRC Biostatistics Unit,
Medical Research Council Centre, Cambridge

ASSESSING CLINICAL TRIALS—
FIRST STEPS

Leading articles,[1-4] correspondence,[5-9] research papers,[10][11] and elementary series[12-14] (see page 1) in the *British Medical Journal* make up a valuable introduction to scientific method and clinical trials. Statistics in Question is an opportunity for revision. The series has a question and answer format with illustrations, and it is in two parts. Assessing clinical trials includes material on medical ethics, consultation, trial size, design, randomisation, observer variability, trial procedures, record sheets, and data checking. The second part deals with statistical methods commonly reported in medical journals and answers questions about their application.

Medical ethics

(1) *Why should the publication of selected series be discouraged if randomised comparison is appropriate?*

—non-randomised studies do not necessarily get the correct answer because of selection bias

—to avoid ethical conflicts randomisation should begin with the first patient[15]

—non-randomised studies lead to rash verdicts

—they do not convince the sceptics

COMMENT

Because of selection bias non-randomised studies can give falsely optimistic[16][17] or even wrong[18] reports of new treatments. Adrenalectomy for essential hypertension—introduced without proper evaluation—was once widely practised but later abandoned because it was of no value.

Again, jejunoileal bypass was introduced without a randomised clinical trial and was widely adopted. Because published reports and their own experience suggested a serious complication rate,[19] Danish surgeons carried out a randomised trial between jejunoileal bypass surgery and medical treatment for patients with morbid obesity.[20] The patients who had bypass surgery

---

Treatments introduced without proper evaluation

1 Adrenalectomy for essential hypertension[18]
2 Adenotonsillectomy in children and young adults[21]
3 Jejunoileal bypass in morbid obesity[20]

---

lost more weight and had a much improved quality of life, though there were complications, some severe. Non-randomised studies had not made their point.

This trial was criticised[22][23] because patients had been deceived—the patients who were randomised to medical treatment were told that the results of liver biopsy contra-indicated surgery. The Danes had faced a dilemma—whether to continue using a treatment about which they had serious doubts or run a randomised trial in which they had to deceive

---

Dilemma

1 Only a randomised trial could convince the Danes
2 Uncritical acclaim by the media had persuaded patients to seek jejunoileal bypass
3 "Informed" consent to medical treatment would probably have been refused
4 Failure to request informed consent is unethical

---

patients. Ethical conflicts could be avoided in future if all procedures, including operations, were evaluated in randomised controlled trials before they were generally adopted.

Smithells *et al*[24] gave periconceptional vitamin supplements to women at high risk of having a baby with a neural-tube defect. One out of 178 infants or fetuses (0·6%) had a neural-tube defect. But among the infants or fetuses of high-risk

---

Vitamins, neural-tube defects, and ethics committees

---

women who were already pregnant or who had refused supplements, 13 out of 260 (5%) had a defect. The study was not randomised because ethics committees at three of the five study centres had refused permission for high-risk women to be assigned randomly to placebo.[25] The poor design of the trial meant that the results were difficult to interpret.[26-29] Selection bias or accidental bias, or both, might account for the different outcomes in the treated and control groups.

Two of the authors wrote[25]: "In our paper we subscribe to no belief, reach no conclusions, and offer four possible interpre-tations...." A less cautious editorial verdict[30] is reason enough to discourage publication of results from selected series when randomisation is appropriate. The pity is that further studies are needed for doctors to know whether or not they can reassure high-risk patients that periconceptional vitamin supplements lessen the risk of neural-tube defect.[28]

(2) When a clinical trial protocol is accepted by the hospital ethics committee is this sufficient guarantee of scientific merit?

—no, protocol review is outside the remit of most ethics committees

—ethics committees usually are only concerned with what is done to the patient

COMMENT

Acceptance of a clinical trial protocol by the hospital ethics committee is not sufficient evidence of scientific value, though it is necessary evidence. Ethical approval was given for the investigation by Smithells *et al* of the possible prevention of neural-tube defects.[24] The control group was self-selected because of either being pregnant or refusing to take periconceptional vitamin supplements. Selection bias could not be dismissed as an explanation for the results, and thus the study had limited scientific value.

Altman (page 3) has discussed the ethical implications of inferior design.[31] But ethics committees are usually only concerned with what is done to the patient,[32] and they are not set up to inquire into the design or size of clinical trials[8][33] (see page 6); it is unusual for a statistician to be on an ethics committee. Protocol review is clearly outside the remit of most ethics committees.

Consultation

(3) What are the five questions a statistician is most likely to ask before advising a doctor on the design of a clinical trial?

What is the precise aim of the investigation?

What is the clinical background?

Are resources limited?

What is the response distribution?

What would be regarded as a clinically important difference between treatments?

COMMENT

The first consultation between the doctor and the statistician should establish the precise aim of the investigation. Trial design is then tailored to fit the right problem. The statistician

> "An approximate answer to the right problem is worth a good deal more than an exact answer to an approximate problem."
>
> John Tukey

will need information about the clinical background, and may ask the doctor for references to recent research articles. Limitation of resources imposes important constraints on the design of a clinical trial. Resources include hospital staff and equipment, time, data processing and secretarial help, finance, and of course patients. The availability of patients is commonly, if unwittingly, overestimated by doctors. The statistician should find out how many suitable patients were referred in, say, the previous six months. There is little point in starting a clinical

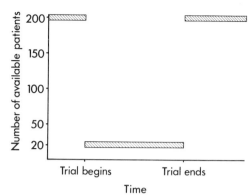

Lasagna's law: the availability of patients is commonly overestimated, even by a factor of 10.

trial whose duration extends beyond the time for which clinical and statistical supervision can be guaranteed.

To determine the number of patients in a clinical trial the statistician must learn something about the response distribution. This could be binary, Gaussian (normal), lognormal, exponential, Poisson, or some other distribution. The doctor may

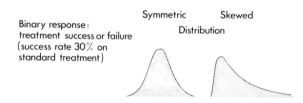

provide this information or it can be deduced from previous research, abstracted from case notes, or obtained in a pilot study.

The doctor must assess the difference between treatments that is clinically important before the statistician can calculate how large the trial should be. Trial size is determined so that if a worthwhile difference exists between treatments the difference will probably be evident, and also statistically significant, in the results.

Pilot studies

(4) Why are pilot studies done?

—to estimate the rate of patient accrual or the variability of treatment outcome

—to test questionnaire, interview, or assessment

—to check that the trial runs smoothly

COMMENT

Pilot studies are devised to estimate patient accrual and the variability of response if this information, which is needed to calculate the size and likely duration of a clinical trial, is not otherwise available (see question 3).

A different type of pilot study is called for when a questionnaire, interview, or assessment scale is used to record information about patients. Form design[34] is not a trivial exercise—content, length, wording, appearance, and layout must be carefully considered. The draft questionnaire should then be tried out (piloted) on a sample of patients to identify language that is difficult to understand or questions that are frankly ambiguous. Do the answers accord with expectation? For example, is height recorded in inches or centimetres?

Startling replies may be elicited by an interviewer. Timing is important in interviews, and it is wise not to rush patients. When a bronchitic patient was asked if he brought up sputum in the morning, he answered, "No," paused, and added as an after-thought, "I swallow it again."

To measure stroke rehabilitation Garraway et al[35] devised a rehabilitation scale. In a series of pilot studies they checked that observers could agree on the interpretation and use of the scale.

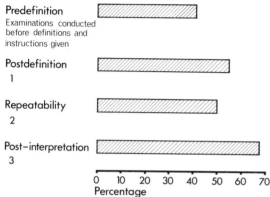

Pilot studies : Clinical assessment of stroke

Predefinition
Examinations conducted before definitions and instructions given

Postdefinition
1

Repeatability
2

Post−interpretation
3

Percentage

Proportion of examinations with total agreement between four examiners (number of examinations equalled 84).

The classic reason for doing a pilot study is to accustom laboratories, hospital staff, and patients to the trial procedures[36] and thus ensure that the experiment runs smoothly. The pilot study mirrors the actual trial in every detail, so that if no amendment is needed the results from patients who have been randomised in the pilot study can be analysed along with the main results.

I am grateful to the editor of *Age and Ageing* for permission to publish the figure on clinical assessment of stroke.

References

1 Anonymous. Statistical errors. *Br Med J* 1977;i:66.
2 Anonymous. Randomised clinical trials. *Br Med J* 1977;i:1238-9.
3 Anonymous. Interpreting clinical trials. *Br Med J* 1978;ii:1318.
4 Anonymous. The case-control study. *Br Med J* 1979;ii:884-5.
5 Pocock SJ. Randomised clinical trials. *Br Med J* 1977;i:1661.
6 Peto R, Doll R. When is significant not significant ? *Br Med J* 1977;ii:259.
7 Anderson TW, Ashley MJ, Clarke EA. Not so double-blind ? *Br Med J* 1976;i:457-8.
8 Newell DJ. Type II errors and ethics. *Br Med J* 1978;ii:1789.
9 Cochrane AL, St Leger AS, Sweetnam P. Emotion and empiricism. *Br Med J* 1979;i:486.
10 Gore SM, Jones IG, Rytter EC. Misuse of statistical methods: critical assessment of articles in *BMJ* from January to March 1976. *Br Med J* 1977;i:85-7.
11 Lionel NDW, Herxheimer A. Assessing reports of therapeutic trials. *Br Med J* 1970;iii:637-9.
12 Swinscow TDV. *Statistics at square one.* London: British Medical Association, 1977.
13 Rose G, Barker DJP. *Epidemiology for the uninitiated.* London: British Medical Association, 1979.
14 Altman DG. Statistics and ethics in medical research. Misuse of statistics is unethical. *Br Med J* 1980;**281**:1182–4.
15 Chalmers TC. When should randomisation begin ? *Lancet* 1968;i:858.
16 Doll R, Peto R. Randomised controlled trials and retrospective controls. *Br Med J* 1980;**280**:44.
17 Colton T. *Statistics in medicine.* Boston: Little, Brown, 1974.
18 Ederer F. The randomised clinical trial. In: Phillips CI, Wolfe JN, eds. *Clinical practice and economics.* London: Pitman, 1977.
19 Anderson B. Research ethics and deception. *Lancet* 1980;i:772.
20 The Danish Obesity Project. Randomised trial of jejunoileal bypass versus medical treatment in morbid obesity. *Lancet* 1979;ii:1255-7.
21 Roydhouse N. A controlled study of adenotonsillectomy. *Lancet* 1969;ii:931-2.
22 Anonymous. Bypassing obesity. *Lancet* 1979;ii:1275-6.
23 Berenbaum MC. Research ethics and deception. *Lancet* 1980;i:772.
24 Smithells RW, Sheppard S, Seller MJ, et al. Possible prevention of neural-tube defects by periconceptional vitamin supplementation. *Lancet* 1980; i:339-40.
25 Smithells RW, Sheppard S. Possible prevention of neural-tube defects by periconceptional vitamin supplementation. *Lancet* 1980;i:647.
26 Kirke PN. Vitamins, neural tube defects, and ethics committees. *Lancet* 1980;i:1300-1.
27 Freed DLJ. Vitamins, neural tube defects, and ethics committees. *Lancet* 1980;i:1301.
28 Raab GM, Gore SM. Vitamins, neural tube defects, and ethics committees. *Lancet* 1980;i:1301.
29 Elwood JH. Possible prevention of neural-tube defects by periconceptional vitamin supplementation. *Lancet* 1980;i:648.
30 Anonymous. Vitamins, neural-tube defects and ethics committees. *Lancet* 1980;i:1601-2.
31 Altman DG. Statistics and ethics in medical research. Study design. *Br Med J* 1980;**281**:1267-9.
32 Thomson IE, French K, Melia KM, et al. Research ethical committees in Scotland. *Br Med J* 1981;**282**:718-20.
33 Altman DH. Statistics and ethics in medical research. III How large a sample ? *Br Med J* 1980;**281**:1336-8.
34 Wright P, Haybittle J. Design of forms for clinical trials (1-3). *Br Med J* 1979;ii:529-30, 590-2, 650-1.
35 Garraway WM, Akhtar AJ, Gore SM, Prescott RJ, Smith RG. Observer variation in the clinical assessment of stroke. *Age Ageing* 1976;**5**:233-40.
36 National Study by the Royal College of Radiologists. A study of the utilisation of skull radiography in 9 accident-and-emergency units in the UK. *Lancet* 1980;ii:1234-6.

ASSESSING CLINICAL TRIALS—
TRIAL SIZE

The size of a clinical trial is decided by balancing statistical considerations—especially the power of the investigation to identify a difference that is clinically important—against practical considerations, such as limitation on time or the availability of patients. In general, the smaller the difference that is judged clinically significant the greater the number of patients needed for a sensible clinical trial.

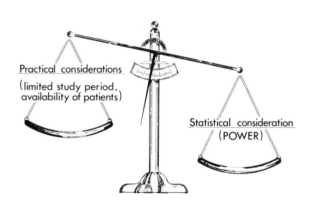

Practical considerations
(limited study period, availability of patients)

Statistical consideration
(POWER)

(5) *The report on a clinical trial concludes that "the difference between treatments is not statistically significant, p > 0·05." Why is it wrong to interpret this as meaning "there is no clinically important difference between the treatments"?*

—inadequate sample size can be the reason for not recognising treatment superiority

—"not statistically significant" does not condemn

—correct interpretation of trial results calls for complete reporting of the statistical methods used to determine trial size, and estimation of confidence intervals

COMMENT

Significance testing is not good statistics. What is needed is estimation. As well as reporting significance levels (p <0·01 versus *"not statistically significant"*), investigators should quote an interval that they are confident covers, or includes, the real treatment difference (see page 15).[1][2] This is no more difficult to do than significance testing, and is more informative. Regrettably, in the medical league confidence intervals have not passed first base.

Reporting only that the difference between treatments is "not statistically significant" may jeopardise correct interpretation of the clinical trial. Freiman *et al*[3] reviewed 71 "negative" binomial trials (a binomial trial is one in which the outcome for an individual patient is categorical, and there are two categories of outcome: treatment success or failure) to determine whether the investigators had studied large enough samples. Forty-five of the

> *Power function:* the confidence with which the investigator can claim that a specified treatment benefit has not been overlooked

trials had less than a 70% chance (POWER) of detecting even a substantial improvement (50%) in cure rate. Estimates of 90% confidence intervals for the true improvement showed that in 34 out of the 71 studies the results were compatible with a 50% difference between cure rates. The authors warned that many treatments labelled as "no different from control" in trials that

> *Aim for 80% power* to detect what is regarded a priori as a realistic, worthwhile treatment difference. Of course, the trial has less power to detect correspondingly smaller differences

use inadequate sample size have not received a fair test. It is wrong to conclude that a non-significant difference rules out the possibility of a worthwhile, or even substantial, clinical difference between treatments (see page 6).[4]

To interpret a clinical trial correctly[5] you need to know the power of the trial to do the job it is intended to do, which is identification of treatment gain, and the trial results need to be reported completely. Complete reporting entails the estimation of confidence intervals. In a survey of 38 clinical trials published from July to December 1977 as original articles in a leading general medical journal, there was no mention of how trial size was determined. What applied in one journal probably applies in others. A survey[6] on the size of randomised controlled trials registered with Union Internationale Contre le Cancer gave more encouraging results. Most investigators used statistical methods to determine trial size. When statistical methods are used it is helpful at least to refer to these in published reports so that readers are aware that statistical considerations weigh heavily in determining trial size. Doctors should be able to absorb good principles in the design of experiments from the very journals they read to keep informed about clinical research and practice.

Wrong decisions in columns 1 and 2 are not too serious, but it is important not to miss a worthwhile treatment difference (column 3).

	①	②	③
REALITY	No difference between treatments	Small difference (clinically insignificant)	Worthwhile treatment difference
CLINICAL TRIAL OUTCOME	5% of trials conclude treatments differ significantly, p<0·05 Direction of difference is fortuitous	A proportion of trials (more than 5% but less than 80%) declare a statistically significant treatment difference	20% of trials find that the difference between treatments is not statistically significant, p>0·05 Direction of treatment difference is probably reliable nevertheless, and so compute confidence interval

*Illustrated for significance level 5%, and trial size chosen to give 80% power for detecting a worthwhile treatment difference.

6) *Fifteen per cent of patients die within one year of admission to hospital for suspected myocardial infarction. Preventing one-third of those deaths would be a major advance. Roughly how many patients are needed for a clinical trial if the doctors want to be 90% sure that a difference between treatments as large as the prevention of one-third of deaths will not be missed (significance level, 5%)?*

—about 2000 patients

COMMENT

About 2000 patients are needed to compare a new treatment against a standard treatment when the critical outcome is prevention of death within a year of admission for suspected myocardial infarction. Only then can doctors be at least 90% sure that a difference between treatments as large as the prevention of one-third of deaths will not be missed.

A randomised double-blind trial compared three drugs—propranolol, atenolol, placebo—in the immediate treatment of suspected myocardial infarction.[7] Only 388 patients were randomised; 259 were given beta-blockers, of whom 36 (14%) died within one year of admission. Of the 129 patients who had received placebo, 19 (15%) died.

The observed difference in death rates at one year was −1%, a point estimate for the true difference. But the estimator has a large standard error because relatively few patients entered the trial.[8 9] The 95% confidence interval for the true difference in death rates is surprisingly wide, from −8% to +7%, and does not exclude the possibility that one treatment or the other prevents one-third of deaths. The interval does not include −10% or +10%, so that prevention of two-thirds of deaths—a dramatic treatment difference—is unlikely. A sufficient number of patients were studied to give a reasonable guarantee against failure to detect only very large treatment differences, such as prevention of two-thirds of deaths. But so large a benefit from beta-blockers, or any other drugs, used in the immediate treatment of suspected myocardial infarction is a priori unlikely.

The published report by Wilcox *et al*[7] was extremely lucid, except in three aspects. There was no statement of the magnitude of treatment effect which the authors considered worth while, no information on how trial size was determined, and no confidence intervals were given. In these omissions the authors are not alone. Elwood and Sweetnam,[10] by comparison, reported on a trial of aspirin after recent myocardial infarction which was designed to detect a 25% reduction in secondary mortality (significance level, 5%). They observed a 17% reduction, which was not statistically significant. Secondary mortality rates were 12·3% and 14·8% in the aspirin and placebo groups respectively; sample size was 1682 patients. For the reduction achieved in

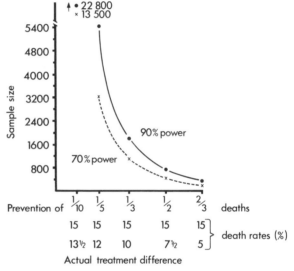

Immediate treatment of suspected myocardial infarction. Beta-blockers versus placebo: significance level 5%.

the trial to have been statistically significant the number of patients (to give 70% power, see figure above) would have had to have been almost double. This puts the power of the trial in perspective. Correctly, the Norwegian report on timolol-induced reduction in mortality after acute myocardial infarction (trial size, 1884 patients) noted that few studies had entered a sufficient number of patients to exclude the possibility of a beneficial effect from beta-blockade being overlooked.[11]

In clinical trials in which the critical outcome is time of death (or time to some other event, such as metastasis) the power of the trial to identify the merits of two treatments depends on how many patients die (or experience the event) rather than on the number of patients entered.[12]

Peto R   Clinical trial methodology

Biomedicine Special Issue 1978; 28: 24-36

Peto[13] has complained that a proliferation of small trials has made it difficult for doctors to know how best to manage suspected myocardial infarction. The review by Chalmers *et al*[14] of 32 comparative studies of anticoagulant treatment, on which Peto comments, did much to clarify the management.

Pocock[15] has given guidelines for calculating sample size in binomial trials, together with worked examples.

References

[1] Altman DG. Statistics and ethics in medical research. VI Presentation of results. *Br Med J* 1980;**281**:1542-4.

[2] Wulff HR. Confidence limits in evaluating controlled therapeutic trials. *Lancet* 1973;ii:969-70.

[3] Freiman JA, Chalmers TC, Smith H, Kuebler RR. The importance of beta, the type II error and sample size in the design and interpretation of the randomised control trial. Survey of 71 "negative" trials. *N Engl J Med* 1978;**299**:690-4.

[4] Altman DG. Statistics and ethics in medical research. III How large a sample? *Br Med J* 1980;**281**:1336-8.

[5] Anonymous. Interpreting clinical trials. *Br Med J* 1978;ii:1318.

[6] Pocock SJ. Size of cancer clinical trials and stopping rules. *Br J Cancer* 1978;**38**:757-66.

[7] Wilcox RG, Roland JM, Banks DC, Hampton JR, Mitchell JRA. Randomised trial comparing propranolol with atenolol in immediate treatment of suspected myocardial infarction. *Br Med J* 1980;**280**:885-8.

[8] Baber NS, Lewis JA. Beta-blockers in the treatment of myocardial infarction. *Br Med J* 1980;**281**:59.

[9] Rose G. Beta-blockers in immediate treatment of myocardial infarction. *Br Med J* 1980;**280**:1088.

[10] Elwood PC, Sweetnam PM. Aspirin and secondary mortality after myocardial infarction. *Lancet* 1979;ii:1313-5.

[11] The Norwegian Multicenter Study Group. Timolol-induced reduction in mortality and reinfarction in patients surviving acute myocardial infarction. *N Engl J Med* 1981;**304**:801-7.

[12] Peto R, Pike MC, Armitage P, *et al*. Design and analysis of randomised clinical trials requiring prolonged observation of each patient. I Introduction and design. *Br J Cancer* 1976;**34**:585-612.

[13] Peto R. Clinical trial methodology. *Biomedicine Special Issue* 1978;**28**:24-36.

[14] Chalmers TC, Matta RJ, Smith H, Kunzler AM. Evidence favouring the use of anticoagulants in the hospital phase of acute myocardial infarction. *N Engl J Med* 1977;**297**:1091-6.

[15] Pocock SJ. Statistical methods in the design and analysis of long-term clinical trials. *Drug treatment and prevention in cerebrovascular disorders*. Amsterdam: Elsevier-North Holland Biomedical Press, 1979:327-42.

ASSESSING CLINICAL TRIALS—
DESIGN I

Treatments may be compared between groups of patients, within-patient simultaneously, or by patients crossing over from one treatment to another. To assess the synergism of propranolol and tienilic acid for the treatment of moderate essential hypertension,[1] for example, it was necessary to study a factorial structure of four treatments: placebo, propranolol, tienilic acid, and tienilic acid combined with propranolol. In a single experiment it is often possible and efficient to investigate the effects and interactions of two or more, perhaps unrelated, treatments by assigning patients to all treatment combinations. Such designs—factorial—should be considered more often.[2]

(7) *What is the advantage of within-patient comparison of treatments?*

—usually far fewer patients are needed

—it can be applied when looking for short-term symptomatic relief of a chronic condition

—disadvantage: beware systemic action and contamination between treatment areas

COMMENT

The advantage of within-patient comparison of treatments is that usually far fewer cases are needed than in a design that calls for patients to be randomised to receive one treatment or another. The reduction in the number of patients comes about without loss of power whenever the responses by an individual in matched sites—for example, right and left eye, right and left scalp—are not as variable as the responses compared between individuals. This is what usually happens in medicine.

Within-patient comparison of treatments should be avoided, however, when treatments can act systemically or when there is the possibility of contamination between treatment areas because bias, unbidden and of unknown extent, intrudes.

Within-patient comparison

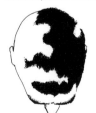

Alopecia areata[3]: treated side should be chosen at random for each patient

Note: by itching or rubbing patient may contaminate the untreated area

Four studies of the induction of hair growth by dinitrochlorobenzene (DNCB) in patients with alopecia areata were reported in the same medical journal.[3-6] All four used within-patient comparison of DNCB versus no treatment. Readers noted[5 7 8]

that DNCB might act systemically in addition to having a local effect; moreover, itching or rubbing the scalp might have contaminated the untreated area. The claims made for DNCB were, if anything, conservative, and DNCB needs to be compared with other treatments and with spontaneous remission. Such a trial would entail randomising patients to one treatment or another.[6]

(8) *What is an example of treatments that must be compared between groups of patients?*

—simple versus radical mastectomy for unilateral breast cancer

COMMENT

The nature of certain treatments precludes within-patient comparison. Simple versus radical mastectomy for stage 1 or 2 unilateral breast cancer can obviously only be compared between groups of patients randomised to one treatment or the other. Simple design principles suffice for many clinical studies. Out of 38 clinical trials reported in the *Lancet* over six months, 28 compared treatments between groups of patients. Mostly two treatments were compared (25 studies). No trial used a factorial design.

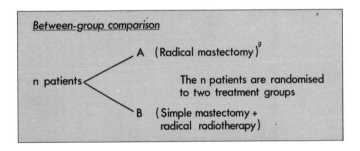

Between-group comparison

n patients

A (Radical mastectomy)[9]

The n patients are randomised to two treatment groups

B (Simple mastectomy + radical radiotherapy)

(9) *What can seriously complicate the analysis of cross-over designs?*

—order effects

—treatment carry-over

COMMENT

An interesting example of a cross-over design was the experiment on how oxprenolol affected stage-fright in musicians.[10] Twenty-four string players each gave two solo performances before an invited audience in the Wigmore Hall. Order effects

```
Cross-over designs (within-patient)

The n patients receive treatments
A,B in the order

‾ ‾ ‾ ‾ ‾ ‾ ‾ ‾ ‾ ‾       Oxprenolol and stage-fright
A(oxprenolol)     B (placebo)     in musicans[10]
              or                   It is usual to randomise patients
‾ ‾ ‾ ‾ ‾ ‾ ‾ ‾ ‾ ‾       to the two orders in such a way
B (placebo)     A (oxprenolol)     as to ensure that half the patients
                                   receive treatments in the order
                                   'A followed by B'

         Note: wash-out periods between treatments — ethical ?
```

(systematic changes between first and subsequent assessments) are not unusual in cross-over trials, and they complicated this example because second performances were rated higher than first performances. An even more serious complication in analysing cross-over designs is when the effect of an earlier treatment persists during one or more subsequent treatments—that is, there is treatment carry-over. Treatment carry-over should be avoided either by inserting a "wash-out period" between treatments or by adopting a different design altogether.

Hills and Armitage[11] wrote an excellent review on the design and analysis of cross-over trials describing how to use pretreatment or base-line observations, how to look for order effects and evidence of treatment carry-over, and how to recognise unbiased treatment comparisons. This paper is essential reading for anyone who is planning a cross-over trial.[12] I suggest, in addition, that doctors consult a statistician about cross-over experiments.

References

1 Pearson RM, Bulpitt CJ, Havard CWH. Biochemical and haematological changes induced by tienilic acid combined with propranolol in essential hypertension. *Lancet* 1979;i:697-9.
2 Peto R. Clinical trial methodology. *Biomedicine Special Issue* 1978;**28**: 24-36.
3 Happle R, Echternacht K. Induction of hair growth in alopecia areata with DNCB. *Lancet* 1977;ii:1002-3.
4 Breuillard F, Szapiro E. Dinitrochlorobenzene in alopecia areata. *Lancet* 1978;ii:1304.
5 Warin AP. Dinitrochlorobenzene in alopecia areata. *Lancet* 1979;i:927.
6 Friedman PS. Dinitrochlorobenzene and alopecia. *Lancet* 1979;i:1412.
7 Anonymous. Alopecia areata. *Br Med J* 1979;i:505.
8 Harrington CJ. Alopecia areata. *Br Med J* 1979;i:1017.
9 Langlands AO, Prescott RJ, Hamilton T. A clinical trial in the management of operable cancer of the breast. *Br J Surg* 1980;**67**:170-4.
10 James IM, Pearson RM, Griffith DNW, Newbury P. Effect of oxprenolol on stage-fright in musicians. *Lancet* 1977;ii:952-4.
11 Hills M, Armitage P. The two-period cross-over clinical trial. *Br J Clin Pharmacol* 1978;**8**:7-20.
12 Anonymous. Planning a cross-over trial. *Lancet* 1979;ii:511.

ASSESSING CLINICAL TRIALS— DESIGN II

At opposite ends of a range are fixed sample size designs and full sequential designs. In the former sample size is determined, or fixed, before the trial begins. In a full sequential design sample size depends in a particular way on the results as they accumulate, and the trial is stopped as soon as a significant difference in treatment is established. Group sequential designs[1] are a compromise between these two approaches. Analyses are planned to coincide with regular trial meetings (at yearly intervals, say). A maximum number of analyses is allowed. At each analysis the decision to stop the trial or to continue is based on correctly applying repeated significance tests to the accumulated data. Doctors should consult a statistician about sequential trials.

Historical comparison alone usually gives insufficient evidence. Non-randomised studies of treatment with anticoagulant drugs during the 1950s and 1960s showed an apparent protective effect (pooled data): the prevention of 53% of deaths after myocardial infarction. The evidence was not sufficient, however, to persuade doctors generally to manage myocardial infarction with anticoagulant drugs. Later, in randomised trials the apparent protective effect of anticoagulant drugs was estimated as preventing 20% of deaths. Note that the bias in the historically controlled studies was of the same order of magnitude as the treatment effect—a grave warning of the errors inherent in historical control series.[2]

In research programmes a treatment is often carried forward from one trial to act as standard or control treatment in the next. Could the patients who have been assigned to this treatment in the earlier study form a historical control group in the later trial? The answer is a qualified yes. Minimum criteria[3] for combining historical and prospective randomised control groups are shown below.

Historical comparison should not take the place of a prospective randomised control group, however.

Sequential trials

(10) *What ethical argument is there against fixed sample size?*

—no patient should receive a treatment that has been established as inferior on the basis of substantial accumulated evidence

—planning interim analyses is therefore a sensible precaution

COMMENT

An ethical argument against fixed sample size is that no patient should receive a treatment that has been found inferior by a substantial accumulation of evidence. A controlled randomised trial[4] of active immunotherapy for stage IIB malignant melanoma was stopped after one year, when only 15 patients had been admitted, because four deaths had occurred in the vaccinated group, three of them after early widespread recurrence of the disease, compared with no deaths in the control group. Unless a formal stopping rule has been defined there may be disagreement about what is sufficient evidence of harm. For this and other reasons there was controversy over the University Group Diabetes Program[5][6] in which treatment by tolbutamide was discontinued.

In the Norwegian multicentre study[7] of mortality after timolol treatment for patients who had had acute myocardial infarction ethical provision was made for confidential and independent interim review of the study information.

It is a sensible precaution to plan interim analyses.

Appropriate adjustment has to be made to the nominal significance level to account for repeated looks at the data. (What do I mean by "nominal significance level"? At each analysis the difference between treatments is tested and if significant at a specified level—the nominal significance level— the trial ends. The nominal significance level is used as a stopping rule, therefore. The rules are worked out in advance of the trial so that overall the sequential plan is associated with an acceptably low risk of a false-positive—that is, of claiming a treatment difference when none exists.) Nominal significance levels are more stringent when there are repeated opportunities for stopping the trial early, so that overall the risk of falsely claiming that one treatment is better than another or better than no treatment remains fixed.

(11) *Why is a fully sequential design often impracticable?*

—treatment results are known too late to limit patient entry

—most fully sequential plans compare only two treatments and assume well-behaved response distributions

—difficult to allow for more than one response variable or to adjust for prognostic factors

—onus on doctors, data-processing staff, and statistician

COMMENT

A fully sequential design is often impracticable when there is a long delay between starting a treatment and its outcome; when there is more than one response variable; when more than two treatments are compared; or when patients have very different prognoses. Even when the outcome is known soon after starting treatment, analysing as soon as the result is known for each patient or patient-pair requires (a) prompt reporting of treatment results to the trial co-ordinator; (b) efficient data processing; (c) the availability of the statistician to update the analysis (unless the doctor enters results on a prepared chart, in which case the treatment code has to be broken).

The doctor, the data-processing staff, and the statistician

have other responsibilities; they cannot spend all their time on a single clinical trial. Together, these reasons explain why fully sequential designs are uncommon despite their ethical appeal.

(12) *If you repeatedly test accumulating data[8] at, say, the 1% nominal significance level, in what way do you alter your chance overall of finding a significant difference?*

—overall the chance of finding a spurious significant difference is increased

COMMENT

If accumulating data are tested repeatedly at a nominal 1% significance level the chance of finding a spurious significant difference is *increased*.[8] For example, if you test for a difference

McPherson K   Statistics: the problem of examining accumulating data more than once

N Engl J Med 1974; 290: 501-2

between two treatments after every 12th patient and intend to stop the trial as soon as the difference is nominally significant at the 1% level, then by the 10th test the effective (type I) error is about 5%—that is, the chance is about 1 in 20 (not 1 in 100 as might be supposed), that a significant difference will

Pocock S J   The size of cancer clinical trials and stopping rules
Br J Cancer 1978; 38: 757-66

be declared even when there is actually no difference between treatments.

Statistical advice should be sought about planning and analysing group sequential trials.

Historical comparison

(13) *Why is the answer "a qualified yes" to the question of whether historical and prospective randomised control groups can be combined?*

—a historical control group—acceptable a priori—is an embarrassment later if comparison of results between historical and prospective randomised control groups approaches significance

COMMENT

If there is an acceptable historical control group the proportion of patients who are randomised to the control arm in the new trial can be reduced. But a historical control group that is acceptable a priori may be an embarrassment later if a comparison of the results between historical and prospective control groups even approaches significance, let alone exceeds conventional levels. A surprisingly large difference (p <0·01) emerged[2] when a treatment group was carried over as control from the fifth

Pocock S J   The combination of randomised and historical controls in clinical trials

J Chron Dis 1976; 29: 175-88

Medical Research Council acute myeloid leukaemia trial to the sixth. In such instances the historical control group must be abandoned, with loss of precision owing to reduced numbers of patients. Pocock[9] reported on 19 (unselected) pairs of consecutive trials in which a combination of historical and prospective randomised groups could have been considered.

Death rate in 1st trial / death rate in 2nd trial

Two-sided significance level (assuming exponential survival)

Consecutive trials: common treatment.[9]

Of the 19 significance levels that compared survival on the same treatment in matched trials, four were embarrassingly significant at the 2% level. Failure to establish bias is not proof that there is no bias.

Thus only qualified approval can be given to the combination of historical and prospective randomised control groups. Seek statistical advice.

(14) *Justify criteria 2, 4, and 5 for combining historical and prospective randomised control groups.*

Minimum criteria for combining historical and randomised control groups[3]

1   Historical control group has received a precisely defined standard treatment that is identical to the treatment for the randomised controls

2   The historical control group must have been part of a recent clinical study with the same requirements for patient eligibility

3   Treatment evaluation should be identical

4   Distribution of important patient characteristics in the historical control group should be comparable with those in new trial

5   Historical trial must have been performed in the same organisation with the same clinical investigators

6   There should be no indicators of differing response between the randomised and historical controls — for example, more rapid accrual, greater enthusiasm for the new trial, better diagnostic aids

2 The group must have been part of a *recent clinical study* with the same requirements for patient eligibility. *Recent* because there may be a time trend in responses or disease characteristics. *Clinical trial membership* because there is a tendency for patients to respond better to treatment in a clinical trial than ordinarily.[10]

4 *The distribution of important patient characteristics* in the historical control group should be comparable with the distribution of those characteristics among patients in the new trial. Otherwise the groups vary obviously in aspects that may determine response. They may be samples from subtly different patient populations.

5 The historical trial must have been performed in the *same organisation* with the *same clinical investigators*—simply because otherwise there may be response differences attributable to organisation.

I am grateful to the editor of the *Journal of Chronic Diseases* for permission to reproduce under question 14 a modified version of the criteria for combining historical and randomised control groups.

References

1 Pocock SJ. The size of cancer clinical trials and stopping rules. *Br J Cancer* 1978;**38**:757-66.

2 Peto R. Clinical trial methodology. *Biomedicine Special Issue* 1978;**28**: 24-36.

3 Pocock SJ. The combination of randomized and historical controls in clinical trials. *J Chron Dis* 1976;**29**:175-88.

4 McIllmurray MB, Embleton MJ, Reeves WG, Langman MJS, Dean M. Controlled trial of active immunotherapy in management of stage IIB malignant melanoma. *Br Med J* 1977;i:540-2.

5 Anonymous. Are antidiabetic drugs dangerous? *Br Med J* 1970;iv:444.

6 Cornfield J. The University Group Diabetes Program. A further statistical analysis of the mortality findings. *JAMA* 1971;**217**:1676-86.

7 The Norwegian Multicenter Study Group. Timolol-induced reduction in mortality and reinfarction in patients surviving acute myocardial infarction. *N Engl J Med* 1981;**304**:801-7.

8 McPherson K. Statistics: the problems of examining accumulating data more than once. *N Engl J Med* 1974;**290**:501-2.

9 Pocock SJ. Randomised clinical trials. *Br Med J* 1977;i:1661.

10 Lennox EL, Stiller CA, Morris Jones PH, Kinnier Wilson LM. Nephroblastoma: treatment during 1970-3 and the effect on survival of inclusion in the first MRC trial. *Br Med J* 1979;ii:567-9.

ASSESSING CLINICAL TRIALS—
WHY RANDOMISE?

The principle of randomisation has been challenged for not being expedient[1]: randomised clinical trials impose a discipline on patient selection and accrual and make ethical considerations explicit and multicentre collaboration necessary if the duration of study is to be limited. What has not been shown is that the principle is ill-founded.[2][3] This article discusses reasons for randomisation and reasons against other schemes of assignment. The next two articles explain simple randomisation—that is, the equivalent to tossing a coin—and restricted randomisation procedures. Randomised clinical trials remain the reliable method for making specific comparisons between treatments.

(15) *What are the purposes of randomisation?*

—to safeguard against selection bias

—as insurance, in the long run, against accidental bias

—as the sinew of statistical tests

COMMENT

Firstly, randomisation is the only safeguard against selection bias: the doctor does not know the treatment assignment for the next patient, and the assignment is maximally unpredictable. There can be neither unwitting nor deliberate selection because there is no identifiable pattern in random allocation. When better results are obtained in one treatment group than in others this may be explained (*a*) by the patient groups not being comparable initially, (*b*) by the superiority of a particular treatment, or (*c*) by a marginal effect of treatment that was enhanced because the distribution of patients to that treatment group was slightly favoured. To eliminate *a* and *c* the investigator must at least be able to defend the method of assigning treatment against the accusation of selection bias. The following example (see figure) cannot be so defended—a comparison of subsequent seizure rates in three groups of children: 87 children whose doctors decided to treat them with long-term anti-

convulsant drugs; 188 children who were not given prophylactic treatment; and 229 children for whom follow-up was allowed to lapse (none of these was given prophylactic treatment). The reason is that allocation of the children to these groups was determined by the paediatrician's assessment and by the stringency of follow-up.

Secondly, randomisation is an insurance in the long run against substantial accidental bias between treatment groups with respect to some important patient variable. The guarantee applies only to large trials; if fewer than 200 patients are randomised a chance imbalance between treatment groups will need careful analysis. In the first Medical Research Council trial of radiotherapy and hyperbaric oxygen for patients with head and neck cancer,[4] 294 patients were randomised to radiotherapy in air or in hyperbaric oxygen. Despite the moderate trial size the treatment groups unfortunately differed in the proportion of patients who had lymph-node metastases in the neck. The hyperbaric oxygen group had the higher proportion of patients —48%—compared with 38% of the 151 patients who had been randomised to treatment in air. A diverse patient population presents a matrix of insufferable complexity.[5] Although randomisation is the surest way through the maze, investigators should still always check that the groups as randomised do not differ with respect to characteristics that are assessed before treatment begins. Nineteen of 28 between-patient trials published in the *Lancet* from July to December 1977 reported making a check

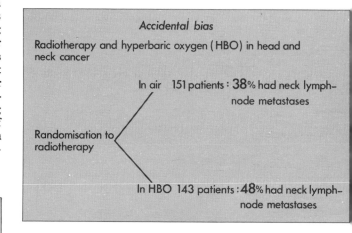

Accidental bias

Radiotherapy and hyperbaric oxygen (HBO) in head and neck cancer

Randomisation to radiotherapy

In air 151 patients: 38% had neck lymph-node metastases

In HBO 143 patients: 48% had neck lymph-node metastases

on how comparable the treatment groups were initially; there was some imbalance in respect of prognostic factors in eight of the 19 studies that made a check. Investigators should not be misled into believing that because randomisation guarantees against accidental bias in the long run that it does so in every instance.

Thirdly, the logical foundation for many statistical tests is the premise that each patient could have received any one of the treatments being compared.

In the survey of 38 clinical trials from the *Lancet* referred to on page 33[6] no trial was uncontrolled, but three trials

Selection bias

Is the question: *Can recurrent febrile convulsions be prevented?* answerable by comparing subsequent seizure rates in

Group 1	87 children for whom, in a paediatrician's judgment, long-term anticonvulsant treatment was appropriate
Group 2	188 children who were given no prophylactic treatment but were followed up adequately
Group 3	229 children who received no prophylactic treatment and were lost to follow-up

relied solely on historical controls. A majority of prospective trials were randomised (22 out of 35), but in only one trial was the randomisation procedure described. Methods of randomisation can be learned only if authors refer to them. Mosteller, Gilbert, and McPeek[7] surveyed controlled randomised trials in myeloma and leukaemia, gastrointestinal cancer, and breast cancer. Only one-third of the 132 articles reported the method of randomisation. Mosteller *et al* suggested that authors should briefly describe how randomisation was performed because only then can the reader properly evaluate the trial. They remarked, "When the randomisation leaks, the trial's guarantee of lack of bias runs down the drain."

(16) *Comment critically on the following non-random assignment schemes: (i) by hospital or surgical team; (ii) by assigning treatments alternately; (iii) by hospital number; (iv) by date of birth.*

(i) liable to serious bias: not only treatment, but also patients' environment and medical supervision differ

(ii) by identifying the treatment for the previous patient doctors can deduce the next assignment

(iii) no safeguard against selection bias

(iv) assignment by date of birth, because it is systematic, invites selection bias;

correlation between morbidity and month of birth

COMMENT

(i) Competitive assignment—that is, when patients referred from different hospitals or by different clinicians receive different treatments—is liable to serious bias. Not only the treatments but also the patients' environment and medical supervision differ,[8] and the latter as much as the former could account for any observed response difference. When the Medical Research Council set up a multicentre trial to compare wound infection rate after major orthopaedic surgery between patients operated on in ultra-clean air and in other theatres, a condition of the trial was that both systems were available in all the trial centres and that the surgical teams operated in both ultra-clean air and in other theatres in random sequence so that, provided the randomisation scheme was adhered to, neither centre nor surgeon would be a source of bias.

Comparison of radical operations in rectal cancer requires that suitable patients are assigned at random to type of operation and that surgical skill is taken into account. A conservative operation is technically more difficult—if it were performed only by specialist teams on selectively referred patients then comparing their results with the outcome of the radical operation by other surgeons could not lead to an unambiguous recommendation of either procedure.

(ii) Alternate assignment of treatments is subject to selection bias if the doctor can identify the treatment for the last patient who entered the trial and so deduce the next assignment. The knowledge may make him defer registration of a particular patient until the treatment he prefers is due for assignment instead of following the unbiased procedure—which is never to register a patient for whom he has a definite treatment preference. Better to limit the population of trial patients than to introduce bias.

Even if the trial treatments are indistinguishable, selection bias can still operate if the doctor knows that the assignment scheme is alternation. All he has to do is guess correctly the treatment for one patient and he can then deduce the treatment for every subsequent patient.

(iii) Assignment by hospital number is unsatisfactory again because there is no safeguard against selection bias. One of the first things that the doctor notices when he looks at a patient's case notes is the hospital number, which is the key to treatment assignment for that patient. The question: "Has forewarning of the treatment group influenced the doctors' decision about whether or not to admit patients to the trial?" will always be asked, and the doubt will linger.

Stead[9] reported that the last digit of the hospital number was used in 1953-5 to assign patients with tuberculosis to three treatments in the ratio 30:30:40. The first and third treatments included streptomycin. Six thousand and nine patients were registered in the trial. Their actual distribution—32% (1898), 26% (1607), 42% (2504)—was significantly different from the target (p < 0.001); the regimen that did not include streptomycin was avoided. Randomisation would have eliminated this subjective element from the selection of treatment.

(iv) Date of birth is almost as obvious a detail in the patient's

Day of birth	Treatment
2, 4, 6, ... 30	Experimental
1, 3, 5, ... 31	Standard

case notes as is hospital number, and so, because it is systematic, assignment by date of birth invites selection bias. There is a second objection—namely, that there may be a correlation

Prophylaxis of postoperative leg vein thrombosis[10]		
Month of birth	Treatment	No of patients
Jan – Apr	Stimulator treatment	88
May – Aug	Low-dose subcutaneous heparin calcium	85
Sept – Dec	Leg exercises only (controls)	122

between morbidity and month of birth.[11] If so, then baseline characteristics as well as treatment differ when patients are allocated by date of birth. It is unnecessary to take this risk. Random assignment may be easily achieved.

Non-random assignment

Surgeon–related variables: eliminated by randomisation, confounded in competitive assignment

Patient : 1 2 3 4 ...

Treatment: *experimental* standard *experimental* standard ...

No 31479
Case notes

References

[1] Gehan E, Freireich E. Non-randomised controls in cancer clinical trials. *N Engl J Med* 1974;**290**:198-203.

[2] Byar DP. Why data bases should not replace randomized clinical trials. *Biometrics* 1980;**36**:337-42.

[3] Meier P. Statistics and medical experimentation. *Biometrics* 1975;**31**: 511-29.

[4] Henk JM, Kunkler PB, Smith CW. Radiotherapy and hyperbaric oxygen in head and neck cancer. *Lancet* 1977;ii:101-3.

[5] Black D. The paradox of medical care. *J R Coll Physicians London* 1979; **13**:57-65.

[6] Gore SM. Assessing clinical trials—design I. *Br Med J* 1981;**282**:1780-1.

[7] Mosteller F, Gilbert JP, McPeek B. Reporting standards and research strategies for controlled trials. Agenda for the editor. *Controlled Clinical Trials* 1980;**1**:37-58.

[8] Irwin TT. Surgeon-related variables. *Lancet* 1978;ii:890.

[9] Stead WW. A suggested change in the method of randomization of patients in therapeutic trials. *Transactions of the 16th conference on the chemotherapy of tuberculosis.* St Louis: Veterans Administration, 1957.

[10] Rosenberg HL, Evans M, Pollock AV. Prophylaxis of postoperative leg vein thrombosis by low dose subcutaneous heparin or preoperative calf muscle stimulation: a controlled clinical trial. *Br Med J* 1975;i:649-51.

[11] Lewis JA. Randomization. *Br Med J* 1975;iii:41.

ASSESSING CLINICAL TRIALS—
SIMPLE RANDOMISATION

Simple randomisation (equivalent to tossing a coin) is the most elementary and probably the most common randomisation procedure in practice (but is not always the best choice: see question 19). Every ploy for guessing the next assignment is equally useless against simple randomisation. Statistical theory determines that the ratio of the number of allocations to each treatment will approach its target as the number of patients increases indefinitely.

Unequal randomisation may be recommended in a wide range of clinical trials in which two treatments are compared: no serious loss of efficiency results from assigning an increased proportion of patients to the experimental treatment (provided the target treatment ratio is not more extreme than 2:1), and there are two advantages—greater clinical experience of the new treatment (compliance, toxicity, etc) is achieved and a more precise estimation of its outcome can be made.

(17) *Use the table of random numbers to determine random treatment assignments for the first 30 patients who enter a clinical trial to compare ordinary spectacles and contact lenses for patients with myopia.*

COMMENT

The first step in determining random treatment assignments is to set up a correspondence between numbers and treatments. Let *odd numbers* correspond to *ordinary spectacles*, and *even numbers* correspond to *contact lenses*. The second step is to determine a convenient systematic way of reading the table of random numbers. The layout reproduced here makes it sensible to use a column of two-digit numbers—for example, 50, 85, 70—and to read down the column.

The third step is to select a starting point. Using a pin I chose *50. For illustration only a fragment from a table of random numbers is reproduced here. Do not use this fragment in practice; consult a more extensive table, select one from the

Table of random numbers

```
25 85  52 40  80 50  80 78  58 42  11 31  85 77  77 25  16 08  54 37
58 73  38 58  78 92  12 38  43 41  31 77  97 3C  33 45  00 17  6C 35
66 04  44 17  00 38  61 37  54 84  38 54  05 96  18 96  20 83  65 29
96 22  27 19  23 83  09 18  22 67  17 31  63 08  80 18  68 08  47 88
29 70  86 38  78 04  51 58  31 92  12 30  98 81  53 09  07 63  23 16

83 86  48 37  00 91  51 91  62 88  04 62  94 63  12 46  51 12  55 22
24 10  43 44  80 33  91 59  46 71  46 72  33 99  13 16  51 34  84 49
26 45  22 19  59 42  70 02* 50 23  78 14  24 19  86 33  37 11  65 36
59 58  24 97  89 51  48 61  85 92  96 83  36 62  06 90  17 23  92 17
14 19  83 76  52 64  91 14  70 66  74 05  47 54  26 81  32 14  91 27

27 70  78 05  51 37  28 77  39 03  63 18  66 74  90 45  23 47  49 80
98 13  78 10  97 38  27 61  27 91  81 70  55 28  35 37  45 76  48 82
94 08  72 66  37 34  44 45  32 26  04 37  80 55  29 88  65 99  63 64
49 76  05 70  91 47  21 85  45 96  57 06  08 49  03 91  19 89  87 10
17 55  25 70  35 57  96 81  90 91  91 05  56 31  55 22  15 63  67 57

57 83  92 42  51 67  49 06  19 44  23 43  39 33  65 52  69 76  98 66
54 36  96 45  91 71  43 43  93 04  71 90  40 81  82 26  56 84  31 32
95 36  83 47  04 07  56 30  59 82  14 82  28 69  27 22  19 47  18 08
61 12  39 28  72 79  97 30  82 43  58 53  40 49  99 71  09 76  60 35
26 27  83 09  88 15  45 34  19 86  67 13  18 50  45 33  02 48  34 58

45 24  50 85  51 89  13 09  85 23  33 26  92 73  47 94  81 86  25 94
44 77  24 50  96 30  18 51  79 05  26 81  87 43  50 71  99 55  32 09
19 79  28 20  23 65  41 96  95 76  81 06  28 11  23 42  78 88  33 42
55 17  44 90  96 22  30 63  61 12  03 95  61 40  29 69  40 05  50 67
73 57  60 29  70 47  76 17  78 45  19 43  68 24  02 39  16 40  86 60

89 02  98 00  17 62  52 94  92 56  80 00  00 26  31 95  24 34  84 41
82 02  00 81  89 86  31 61  31 23  38 70  16 15  93 06  97 44  33 63
52 01  93 94  50 55  19 39  99 45  33 41  40 40  71 54  95 11  19 13
64 80  82 89  45 39  32 76  89 53  80 65  44 77  23 81  89 46  93 31
78 83  74 73  25 33  78 96  68 49  40 11  35 36  17 50  41 41  48 02

                                        **
16 71  31 07  82 88  89 96  44 21  88 20  22 77  23 29  83 14  38 06
98 90  44 87  42 03  23 23  87 14  30 08  25 17  46 51  03 58  46 62
34 95  90 75  63 46  67 53  13 59  91 93  58 51  43 69  78 88  37 65
30 27  22 59  07 85  95 97  61 29  31 56  28 11  26 71  99 13  31 37
00 08  48 54  49 72  89 48  59 49  15 41  70 48  69 97  49 77  29 22

33 57  45 38  37 68  28 69  03 29  50 80  59 48  61 60  85 08  65 40
54 34  43 44  14 00  94 50  67 57  68 15  08 20  25 55  19 37  75 38
74 21  68 80  20 75  39 51  58 77  39 47  93 74  54 29  26 18  18 59
65 09  82 46  75 80  58 91  62 39  49 97  01 57  90 83  42 44  47 34
10 43  48 61  60 65  96 45  17 33  03 50  78 26  85 72  61 01  67 75

01 94  95 31  34 40  15 77  57 25  94 76  77 95  34 61  57 80  84 91
57 72  84 03  52 33  45 45  54 58  76 24  11 70  47 64  31 34  00 52
85 89  47 95  04 23  30 42  91 63  50 27  31 88  37 53  93 46  14 34
11 43  25 72  26 18  52 81  68 53  65 65  62 77  29 63  81 17  21 73
73 62  52 21  84 78  63 17  45 28  35 53  90 79  80 43  87 65  80 44

55 91  18 37  95 71  45 13  16 10  65 76  74 52  87 59  10 93  00 48
26 40  72 27  23 11  80 68  17 82  54 90  09 34  15 03  92 54  52 71
28 53  58 92  62 13  56 50  36 18  96 48  96 31  03 67  94 99  60 37
39 70  30 58  87 42  52 62  06 97  20 58  52 63  22 29  13 57  34 10
75 78  85 97  01 92  55 74  85 83  02 12  07 93  32 86  31 21  41 32
```

several pages of random numbers therein, and choose a starting point on that page. These selections need not be made in a strictly random fashion—the use of a pin is not unusual, for example—but steps one, two, and three should be fully documented so that the randomisation can be followed or continued by a colleague. Randomisation by flipping a coin or tossing a die is not recommended because it cannot be checked or reproduced.

The fourth step is to make the treatment assignments according to the system defined above. Thus I assign patients 1 to 30 as follows:

Treatment: ordinary spectacles or CONTACT LENSES

ordinary, ordinary, ordinary, ordinary, ordinary

Even if the last 5 patients were assigned to ordinary spectacles the probability remains ½ that the next patient receives ordinary spectacles (every guessing strategy is equally useless)

Patient	Random number	Assignment
1	50	CONTACT LENSES
2	85	ordinary spectacles
3	70	CONTACT LENSES
4	39	ordinary spectacles
5	27	ordinary spectacles
6	32	CONTACT LENSES
7	45	ordinary spectacles
8	90	CONTACT LENSES
9	19	ordinary spectacles
10	93	ordinary spectacles
11	59	ordinary spectacles
12	82	CONTACT LENSES
13	19	ordinary spectacles
14	85	ordinary spectacles
15	79	ordinary spectacles
16	95	ordinary spectacles
17	61	ordinary spectacles
18	78	CONTACT LENSES
19	92	CONTACT LENSES
20	31	ordinary spectacles
21	99	ordinary spectacles
22	89	ordinary spectacles
23	68	CONTACT LENSES
24	44	CONTACT LENSES
25	87	ordinary spectacles
26	13	ordinary spectacles
27	61	ordinary spectacles
28	59	ordinary spectacles
29	03	ordinary spectacles
30	67	ordinary spectacles

The above random assignment results in nine patients only being given contact lenses out of the first 30 who are registered in the trial. Such an unequal allocation is not unusual when simple randomisation is used to assign treatments to a small number of patients.

If there were only 30 patients in the trial then in practice the above assignment would be rejected in its entirety and the simple randomisation procedure repeated until a more balanced assignment was achieved—acceptable limits of imbalance would usually be predetermined—[12:18], say—or a method of restricted randomisation would be used (see "Restricted randomisation," page 44). To repeat the simple randomisation continue reading down the same column—58, 62, 17—and then from the top of the next column—42, 41, 84—down to 91, 44, 04; this second randomisation assigns contact lenses to 13 patients, ordinary spectacles to 17—a more respectable divide, which would be retained as a practical assignment if the target number of patients for the trial were only 30.

Suppose that the instruction had been to assign patients to one of three treatments: ordinary spectacles, bifocal spectacles, or contact lenses. A correspondence between two-digit numbers and treatments has to be established. One simple scheme is:

    00-29   ordinary spectacles
    30-59   bifocal spectacles
    60-89   contact lenses
    90-99   IGNORE

Notice that it is convenient to use only the numbers 00-89, which are divided into three sets of 30 numbers each. Equal weight is thereby given to each treatment. The numbers 90-99 are ignored.

(18) *Reassign the 30 patients in question 17 in the ratio 3:2— contact lenses versus ordinary spectacles.*

—three out of five patients should be assigned to contact lenses

—set up a correspondence between numbers and treatments

COMMENT

Three out of five patients should be assigned to contact lenses. Let the correspondence between two-digit numbers and treatments be:

    00-59   contact lenses
    60-99   ordinary spectacles

Read down columns of two-digit random numbers. I begin at **22, 25, 58. Treatment assignments for the first 30 patients are as follows:

Patient	Random number	Assignment
1	22	CONTACT LENSES
2	25	CONTACT LENSES
3	58	CONTACT LENSES
4	45	CONTACT LENSES
5	70	ordinary spectacles
6	59	CONTACT LENSES
7	08	CONTACT LENSES
8	93	ordinary spectacles
9	01	CONTACT LENSES
10	78	ordinary spectacles
11	77	ordinary spectacles
12	11	CONTACT LENSES
13	31	CONTACT LENSES
14	62	ordinary spectacles
15	60	ordinary spectacles
16	74	ordinary spectacles
17	09	CONTACT LENSES
18	96	ordinary spectacles
19	52	CONTACT LENSES
20	07	CONTACT LENSES
21	77	ordinary spectacles
22	30	CONTACT LENSES
23	96	ordinary spectacles
24	08	CONTACT LENSES
25	81	ordinary spectacles
26	63	ordinary spectacles
27	99	ordinary spectacles
28	19	CONTACT LENSES
29	62	ordinary spectacles
30	54	CONTACT LENSES

The actual assignment—contact lenses 16 patients: ordinary spectacles 14 patients—is tolerably close to the target of 3:2.

(19) When are there disadvantages in using simple randomisation?

—if the eventual trial size is less than 100 patients

—in multicentre trials

—if interim analyses are planned

COMMENT

In trials of fewer than 100 patients simple randomisation may too easily result in gravely unequal treatment numbers. One reason why the randomisation list should be prepared in advance of the trial is so that a discrepant allocation can be spotted and an alternative randomisation selected with a more balanced assignment (advice which is pragmatic, not puristic).

Small trials

The probability of discrepant allocation when 30 patients are assigned by simple randomisation to two treatments is as follows:

Group sizes		Probability
15	15	0·144
14	16	0·271
13	17	0·223
12	18	0·161
11	19	0·102
10	20	0·056
9	21	0·027
8	22	0·011
7	23 or worse	0·005

The probability of discrepancy [11,19] or worse is 0·20

The investigator who adopts simple randomisation for a small trial cannot forestall a chance imbalance on some major factor affecting prognosis. For example, in a trial to compare home treatment with sanatorium treatment in tuberculosis patients in Madras[1] 37 (46%) out of 80 patients who were randomised simply to drug treatment at home had extensive cavitation

compared with only 22 (28%) of the 79 patients given the same treatment in a sanatorium. Later trials stratified by this important variable—that is, they ensured that patients with extensive cavitation were represented equally in all treatment groups and, likewise, that the proportion of patients with lesser cavitation was also similar across all treatment groups.

A single simple randomisation list cannot be recommended for multicentre trials because even when treatment numbers are balanced over the trial as a whole patients may be unequally allocated between treatments at individual hospitals, which is irksome to those hospitals and seems careless when the trial is reported.

Interim analyses may include far fewer numbers of patients than the eventual report. Although simple randomisation may serve well for the trial as a whole, treatment numbers or the distribution of patient characteristics may be decidedly unequal at the first and perhaps later interim analyses, which become handicapped as a consequence. The problem of imbalance on some patient variable at interim analysis occurs with other randomisation schemes too. A trial of neutron treatment in patients with head and neck cancer is in progress at the Medical Research Council Cyclotron Unit in Edinburgh. Patients are stratified by the site of the primary tumour and by the presence or absence of nodes before restricted randomisation (see "Restricted randomisation") to neutron or photon treatment. At the first and second interim review treatment groups were well balanced on these important prognostic variables (as intended) but the ratio of men to women patients was different on the two treatment arms at the first analysis and had not resolved by the second review.

Interim analyses

Imbalance between treatment numbers or unequal distribution of patient characteristics, or both

	1st review (Aug 1979)		2nd review (Oct 1980)	
	Photon	Neutron	Photon	Neutron
No of men	15	25	22	35
No of women	15	3	23	9
Total	30	28	45	44

The disadvantages inherent in simple randomisation show the need for methods of restricted and stratified randomisation, which are discussed next.

I am grateful to Professor David F Kerridge, University of Aberdeen, for permission to reproduce the table of random numbers from *Tables and Formulae*. I am also grateful to Professor W Duncan and Miss G R Kerr for permission to mention the trial of neutron treatment in patients with head and neck cancer.

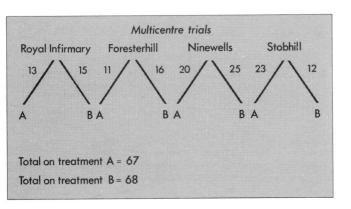

Multicentre trials

Royal Infirmary Foresterhill Ninewells Stobhill

13 / 15 11 / 16 20 / 25 23 / 12

A B A B A B A B

Total on treatment A = 67
Total on treatment B = 68

Reference

[1] Tuberculosis Chemotherapy Centre, Madras. A concurrent comparison of home and sanatorium treatment of pulmonary tuberculosis in South India. *Bull WHO* 1959;**21**:51-144.

ASSESSING CLINICAL TRIALS— RESTRICTED RANDOMISATION

Restricted randomisation[1-3] is recommended when investigators want to ensure that the numbers of patients allocated to each treatment are approximately equal in the trial as a whole or in important subgroups of patients, or both. Corresponding methods, in order of increasing complexity, are the method of random permuted blocks, stratified randomisation, and minimisation. These are discussed here, but Zelen[1] has given a fuller account. He is also responsible for a new design— randomised consent[4]—which is also discussed.

The method of random permuted blocks is easy to use. In the trial as a whole it guarantees that the numbers allocated to each treatment are equal after every block of so many patients has entered.

Stratification[1] by one factor (perhaps two) that is known to affect prognosis is a safeguard against a chance imbalance between treatment groups with respect to an important variable —for example, the extent of cavitation in tuberculosis or axillary node disease in breast cancer. Stratification, especially in small trials, is recommended so long as the randomisation is still simple to operate. One method is to devise a separate list for each stratum by the method of random permuted blocks—that is, consult different lists according to the extent of cavitation for a patient with tuberculosis.

Stratified randomisation may also be useful in multicentre trials when it is important to avoid treatment imbalance in individual hospitals as well as in the trial as a whole. One way of doing this when there are many centres is to prepare randomisation lists for the trial as a whole, monitor the imbalance in individual hospitals, and intervene to restore the balance within a hospital before the assignments there get too far out of line.

Minimisation,[3] as the word implies, is a method of random assignment that minimises the marginal imbalance in the numbers of patients allocated to different treatments over several (two or more) factors known to affect prognosis, one of which may be hospital in a multicentre study. The method avoids the limitations of stratified randomisation (see question 21) but has a similar purpose. It works this way: a measure of imbalance is calculated over the set of prognostic factors describing the new patient, who is then most probably, but not invariably, assigned to the treatment that minimises the overall imbalance.

Randomised consent designs[4] have a different rationale: (a) to limit the number of patients to whom a full and perhaps distressing explanation is given of the purpose of a randomised trial; and (b) to encourage doctors to participate in clinical trials. Some doctors fear that informed consent—as regulated by the Federal Government in the United States, for example— destroys their patients' hope and confidence. These doctors refer no patients or only selected ones for inclusion in clinical trials. Zelen[4] proposed that all eligible patients should be randomised to a "seek consent" or a "do not seek consent" group. The latter receives the standard treatment; the former group is asked to give informed consent to the experimental treatment. Comparison is made between *groups as randomised*, though the "seek consent" group will have a proportion of patients who received the standard treatment—because they so decided after the trial had been fully explained, or because their

doctor elected not to confront them with a traumatic explanation. These designs are new and therefore uncommon in published reports.

Random permuted blocks

(20) *The doctor has realised that the randomisation plan is to make the numbers allocated to each treatment equal after every block of four patients has entered (see figure). What problem occurs when he can identify the treatments given to the first three patients in any block?*

—selection bias because the treatment for every fourth patient can be deduced

COMMENT

The method of random permuted blocks works well provided that the doctor does not guess the block length (four in my example) and cannot identify the treatments that have been assigned to previous patients in the block. If he can identify the first three assignments and realises that the block length is four then he knows that the last patient in the block must

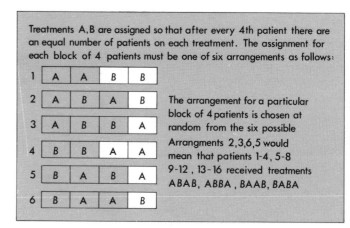

Treatments A,B are assigned so that after every 4th patient there are an equal number of patients on each treatment. The assignment for each block of 4 patients must be one of six arrangements as follows:

1	A	A	B	B
2	A	B	A	B
3	A	B	B	A
4	B	B	A	A
5	B	A	B	A
6	B	A	A	B

The arrangement for a particular block of 4 patients is chosen at random from the six possible Arrangments 2,3,6,5 would mean that patients 1-4, 5-8 9-12 , 13-16 received treatments ABAB, ABBA , BAAB, BABA

Permuted block randomisation: block length 4. (a) There are 24 arrangements of 3 A's and 3 B's, corresponding to block length 6. (b) Tables of random permutations[5] should be used if there are too many arrangements to list—when block size exceeds six patients, for example. (c) In single-centre trials avoid small block size—choose a block length of 10 or more patients, or vary block length randomnly.

receive the treatment that makes things equal. Selection bias then becomes a problem, especially if the block length is short (equal treatment numbers after every second or every fourth or every sixth patient). In my example selection bias could affect decisions about as many as one-third of the trial patients. Clearly the statistician should not tell the doctor what the block length is and will often take the precaution of varying block length randomly to make the detective work more difficult.

There are other methods of restricted randomisation that are not liable to selection bias even when treatments are unmasked. They entail simple randomisation when the discrepancy between the numbers of patients in each treatment group is small but give greater weight (probability $\frac{2}{3}$, say) to the treatment group that is deficient in numbers when the deficiency goes beyond a predefined limit. Descriptions have been given by Zelen[1] and Efron.[2]

Stratification

(21) *Why is excessive stratification self-defeating?*

—deters participation in a clinical trial

—results in too many strata with too few patients

—administrative complexity leads to errors

Strata: clinical state at entry to trial	Treatment numbers		
	Disodium cromoglycate	Sulphasalazine	Combination
Clinical attack	5	5	6
Clinical remission			
Inflamed on sigmoidoscopy	7	7	8
Not inflamed on sigmoidoscopy	25	25	19
Total	37	37	33

Stratified randomisation: comparison of disodium cromoglycate and sulphasalazine as maintenance treatment for ulcerative colitis[6] (patients allocated by restricted randomisation in each stratum).

COMMENT

A chance imbalance occurring between treatment groups on factors unrelated to the prognosis is of no practical importance whatsoever. It is only worth considering stratification by variables that are known to affect prognosis. These are usually few. Overzealous stratification is a humbug—factor levels must be multiplied (not added) to yield the total number of subgroups. Even three prognostic factors, such as tumour size, axillary node disease, and menstrual status in breast cancer, each at three levels—tumour size: $\leqslant 2$ cm, 3-4 cm, $\geqslant 5$ cm; axillary node disease: not diseased, mobile, matted nodes; menstrual status: premenopause, menopausal, postmenopause—yield $3 \times 3 \times 3 = 27$ subgroups of patients. For each of these a separate restricted randomisation list must be consulted. Worse still, the distribution of patients is unlikely to be even, so that many strata will include so few patients that the restricted randomisation procedure does not come into play—for example, balancing treatment numbers after every sixth patient is not effective in strata with fewer than six patients. And so treatment numbers need not be equal, even in the trial as a whole. Excessive stratification is therefore self-defeating.

Besides, an adjustment may be made retrospectively at the analysis to cope with moderate differences between treatment groups in relation to a variable—age at menarche, for example—that was not considered important before as a predictor of survival.

Minimisation

(22) *The figure below shows the assignment so far: 60 patients with breast cancer have been randomised to simple mastectomy + radiotherapy or to radical mastectomy. Patient 61 is premenopausal and has a tumour that is 5 cm in size and positive axillary nodes. Which treatment assignment leads to the least imbalance over the relevant (shaded) prognostic factors?*

—simple mastectomy + radiotherapy

—patient 61 is assigned to this treatment with probability greater than $\frac{1}{2}$ but less than 1—that is, the probable assignment is weighted in favour of simple mastectomy + radiotherapy

	Menstrual status		Tumour size (cm)			Nodes	
Treatment	Pre-menopause	Post-menopause	$\leqslant 2$	3-4	$\geqslant 5$	Negative	Positive
Simple mastectomy + radiotherapy (n=30)	8	22	4	14	12	17	13
Radical mastectomy (n=30)	7	23	5	12	13	14	16
Total No of patients	15	45	9	26	25	31	29

Balancing treatments over several prognostic factors
Assignment so far...

Patient 61 is pre menopausal, has tumour size 5cm and positive nodes

The second figure shows that of the 15 premenopausal patients who have been treated so far, seven have undergone radical mastectomy. By assigning patient 61 also to radical mastectomy the numbers of such patients would be made the same in both treatment groups. On the other hand, assignment to simple mastectomy+radiotherapy is preferred to minimise the imbalance between treatment groups in respect both of patients who have a large tumour and of patients with positive nodes.

A trivial measure of overall imbalance would be the number of votes for and against each treatment. Simple mastectomy+

Patient description	Assignments so far		Favoured assignment for patient 61
	Simple mastectomy + radiotherapy	Radical mastectomy	
Premenopause	8	7	Radical mastectomy
Tumour size ⩾5cm	12	13	Simple mastectomy + radiotherapy
Positive nodes	13	16	Simple mastectomy + radiotherapy

radiotherapy wins because it has two votes. But this measure can be criticised because it does not take into account that an imbalance of 13 versus 16 is in more need of correction than one of 8 versus 7. Thus if patient 61 were assigned to radical mastectomy the overall imbalance would then be $(8-8)+(12-14)+(13-17)=-6$, compared with 0 if simple mastectomy+radiotherapy were selected. This more sensitive criterion also favours simple mastectomy+radiotherapy. What happens next is that patient 61 has a high chance—probability $\frac{3}{4}$, say—of being assigned to simple mastectomy+radiotherapy but could nevertheless still be randomised to radical mastectomy—probability $\frac{1}{4}$—which exaggerates the imbalance. It is important to retain the random element—assignment with a probability of less than 1—to avoid selection bias.

Randomised consent design

(23) *Identify at least two disadvantages of randomised consent designs.*

—**difficulty in making the trial double-blind**

—**only patients in the "seek consent" group know that they are taking part in a clinical trial**

—**doctors may be more persuasive in presenting information about the new treatment to some types of patients than to others**

Randomised consent designs[4] have several limitations. The first is that it is difficult to arrange for such a trial to be double-blind, since membership in the group is revealed by whether or not the patient was asked for informed consent to the experimental treatment. The second difference between the randomised groups is that the patients in one group know that the outcome of their treatment is of special interest to doctors. This knowledge may influence compliance with treatment or the patients' reporting of disease status, and so bias the comparison between treatments. A third problem comes when the results are analysed

if the proportion of patients who agree to the experimental treatment differs between subgroups. The different proportions of patients need not truly reflect whether the experimental treatment was acceptable to different types of patients but may depend on how persuasively doctors presented the information about the new treatment. The problem is especially tricky if the experimental treatment actually benefits some subgroups but is inferior to the standard treatment in others. This interaction could be hidden in the trial results if doctors, guessing it correctly, advocated the experimental treatment strongly only for those patients in whom they expected the most benefit. When the trial came to be analysed the "seek consent" group would have the better results, but it would be noted that in some subgroups a high proportion of patients' refused the experimental treatment. There can be no clear interpretation of the reasons for refusal; refusal is not necessarily an indictment of the experimental treatment, but it may be. Randomised consent designs are useful only when a consistently high proportion of patients in the "seek consent" group accepts the experimental treatment.

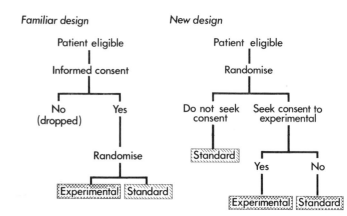

Telephone randomisation

(24) *What precautions should be taken if the mechanism for random assignment is (i) sealed envelopes; (ii) coded phials (supplied by the hospital pharmacy or a drug company, for example); (iii) central randomisation office (telephone randomisation)?*

(i) **beware of transparent envelopes;**

keep a register of trial patients by name, date of registration, and trial number

(ii) **ensure that the phials are identical in shape, instruction label, seal, and contents;**

the code should give no clue as to the contents of the phial—avoid labels such as "treatment A" or "treatment B";

give expiry date and batch number

(iii) **the best safeguard against the curious and the ingenious;**

avoid delay by manning the randomisation office during agreed hours;

give written confirmation after telephone randomisation

(i) If the random assignments are in sealed numbered envelopes the trial co-ordinator must ensure that the next assignment cannot be read by holding the envelope up to the light. The decision to register a patient in the clinical trial should be made before the treatment is revealed: the decision is appropriate only if the doctor is prepared for that patient to receive any one of the trial treatments, otherwise assignment is contraindicated. One way to defend the integrity of the randomisation scheme is for a trial co-ordinator to hold the sealed envelopes and keep a log of registered patients so that a one-to-one correspondence is set up between patient and sealed numbered assignment. Of course, a master randomisation list is also held.

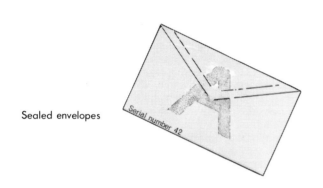

Sealed envelopes

Serial number 42

(ii) When coded phials are prepared in advance by the hospital pharmacy (or elsewhere) it is important that the contents of the phials are indistinguishable and that the phials are identical in shape, instruction label, and seal. The code should identify the phial as for use by patient number 4 in study week 1, say, and should give no clue, however vague, as to the contents of

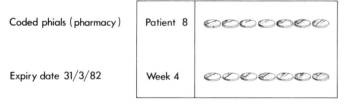

| Coded phials (pharmacy) | Patient 8 | ⬭⬭⬭⬭⬭⬭⬭ |
| Expiry date 31/3/82 | Week 4 | ⬭⬭⬭⬭⬭⬭⬭ |

the phial. If two treatments are compared, do not describe these on the phials as treatments A, B since the doctor then has a 50% chance of guessing correctly the assignment for

every patient—all he has to do is match code A to the correct treatment. It is also important that if the labelled phials are released by the pharmacy or by a drug company to individual doctors that advice is given about the expiry date of the drugs and about batch numbers if more than one batch has been supplied. It would be most unfortunate if a delay in starting the trial meant that some patients received out-of-date medicines. It is also important to register trial patients formally, either locally or with a central co-ordinator, so that there is no opportunity for substituting one patient for another.

(iii) A central randomisation office removes from individual hospitals or doctors the chore of administering the randomisation and safeguards the scheme from the curious and the ingenious. Telephone randomisation works well provided (a) that the

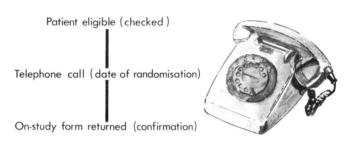

Central randomisation office (telephone randomisation)

Patient eligible (checked)

Telephone call (date of randomisation)

On-study form returned (confirmation)

randomisation office is manned during well-publicised and agreed hours so that doctors are not kept waiting when they telephone with details about an eligible patient; and (b) that the clerk notes the patient's name, the hospital, the name of the doctor who makes the call, and checks the patient's eligibility for the trial. The treatment assignment will then be given out for that patient and registered by the clerk. The date of the telephone call is the date of registration in the trial. Details are then confirmed in writing by the doctor, who submits an on-study form for the patient.

References

[1] Zelen M. The randomisation and stratification of patients to clinical trials. *J Chron Dis* 1974;**27**:365-75.
[2] Efron B. Forcing a sequential experiment to be balanced. *Biometrika* 1971;**58**:403-17.
[3] White SJ, Freedman LS. Allocation of patients to treatment groups in a controlled clinical study. *Br J Cancer* 1978;**37**:434-47.
[4] Zelen M. A new design for randomized clinical trials. *N Engl J Med* 1979;**300**:1242-5.
[5] Schwartz D, Flamant R, Lellouch J. Randomisation. *Clinical trials*. London: Academic Press, 1980.
[6] Willoughby CP, Heyworth MF, Piris J, Truelove SC. Comparison of disodium cromoglycate and sulphasalazine as maintenance therapy for ulcerative colitis. *Lancet* 1979;i:119-22.

ASSESSING CLINICAL TRIALS—
BETWEEN-OBSERVER VARIATION

"Poor repeatability implies poor validity"[1]—as in epidemiology, so too in clinical trials. Unless a satisfactory answer can be given to the question: How reproducible are results by the same observer?—for example, on a second occasion or on repeat specimens—the assessment should be rejected in favour of another that measures the same thing but which is of proved repeatability. This rule applies in pathology (selecting assays or staining techniques), radiography, ultrasonography, and other subjects, and even to recording clinical signs. A sign carries no information if doctors assess it differently when re-examining the patient.

Even when the field has been narrowed to repeatable measurements that are also valid—that is, they measure what they purport to measure—the problem of between-observer variation remains. A doctor eliciting signs in respiratory disease,[2] a neurologist making a tentative diagnosis of multiple sclerosis,[3] a geriatrician assessing stroke rehabilitation,[4] or an anaesthetist determining fitness for operation[5] is each making a judgment that might be made differently by another doctor. Variation between observers in a clinical trial can seriously compromise the research findings. The worst example is when all patients who are given drug A are assessed by one doctor, while a different doctor evaluates patients having drug B. The outcome of such a trial is completely uninformative because any result can be accounted for by the difference between observers rather than between drugs. To avoid the problem one can arrange for the same observer to assess all the patients, but this is not always practicable because of considerations such as the efficient running of wards and clinics and the doctors' duty rota. At least ensure that the same observer makes serial assessments on a given patient, and when there is more than one observer identify which observer assesses which patient (observer code).

(25) *How can variation between observers be reduced?*

—**use an expert panel or reference laboratory**

—**compare rival assessment schemes in a pilot study**

—**find out in what way the observer may be biased**

—**train observers**

—**standardise the techniques and criteria for making judgments**

—**consider: how serious is the disagreement?**

—**randomise patients to observer**

—**defer the trial**

—**appoint an assessor to the research team**

COMMENT

Observer variation may be tackled by appointing a specialist panel to review all trial diagnoses—pathological, radiological, scintigraphic, etc. Ideally this evaluation should be done before randomising patients to treatment to avoid retrospective exclusion. Pathological, haematological, or biochemical trial results may often be submitted to a reference laboratory. Such results should of course be reviewed blind, with no knowledge of the treatment assignment.

Another approach is to compare rival assessment schemes in a pilot study to find which scheme leads to the greatest consensus among observers. Thus Oldham[6] showed that classifying chest radiographs by the presence or absence of tuberculosis or by the clinical significance of the shadows could be repeated reliably more often than classifying them by disease activity or inactivity. When designing this type of pilot study remember that patients who have shown dramatic improvement or appreciable deterioration will be correctly identified by most observers on almost any criteria. It is the patients who have shown a partial response who are most difficult to classify. A good assessment scheme leads to consensus on these patients also.

Be suspicious of any rating—such as behaviour rating in schizophrenia[7] by nurses on a linear scale (scored 0 to 10)—which has not been studied for observer variation. Remember also that consensus alone is not enough: there must be evidence that the assessment is a reliable diagnostic test or measure of recovery. For example, speech therapists independently assessed school entrants[8] to whom doctors had given a simple speech screening test. In the field trial an accuracy rate of 92% for the 438 children was reported, and the referral rate by the doctors was 14%. Speech therapists subsequently observed or treated 44 children: nine of them had passed the simple screening test.

Understanding in what way the observer may be biased may reduce observer variation. It has been suggested that an unconscious bias towards lowering or raising a patient's blood pressure is created by making an arbitrary division between normal and high blood pressure[9]—likewise the awareness of risk factors, such as obesity, or a threshold for clinical trial entry. Wilson et al[5] estimated the degree of optimism and pessimism shown by 10 anaesthetists in assessing whether patients were fit for elective surgery. Another aspect of measurement error is that sometimes an observer may prefer even values when instruments such as manometers and applanation tonometers are marked off at even pressures; and a preference for the terminal digits 0 and 5 has also been noted. The tendency to avoid the extremes on any scale is illustrated by this example (for which I thank Dr S J Daldry): a class of 105 statistics undergraduates were asked to write down an integer in the range 0 to 9. The histogram below is certainly not consistent with uniform preference. In particular, the numbers 0 and 9 were avoided.

Training and practice reduce inter-observer variation. In the clinical assessment of stroke[4] observer agreement was increased from 55% at the first attempt after receiving instruction and definition to 68% at the third test (estimated from 84

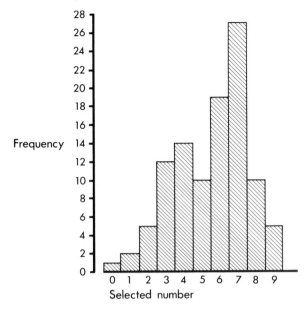

105 undergaduates select a number in the range 0-9

Frequency / Selected number

Diagnostic classification for multiple sclerosis for 149 patients by two neurologists (observers)						
Diagnostic class	Neurologist B				Total	Proportion
	Certain	Probable	Possible	Doubtful		
Neurologist A — Certain	38	5	0	1	44	0·30
Probable	33	11	3	0	47	0·32
Possible	10	14	5	6	35	0·23
Doubtful	3	7	3	10	23	0·15
Total	84	37	11	17	149	
Proportion	0·56	0·25	0·07	0·11		

assessments). Observers who differ in experience are likely to differ systematically in their assessments on that account. Reports from painstaking assessors will be subject to less random error.

Inter-observer variation can be limited by standardisation—that is, by adhering to particular routines, such as agreed guidelines for physical examinations and selection of diagnostic tests, specified reagents for use in laboratory assessments, and carefully worded questions asked in a given order. In ophthalmology ocular tension is measured systematically first in the right eye and then in the left; visual acuity is measured in standard lighting conditions and at a prescribed distance from the Snellen chart; and patients are encouraged to read as far down the chart as they can. The standardisation of blood pressure measurement has been well described[9] but has not been adequately reported in medical journals. Two-thirds of 96 papers relating to blood pressure that had been published in four prestigious general medical journals failed to report on one or more of the following[10]: the type of equipment used; the diastolic end-point; the number of readings per measure-

> The case for standardisation has not been made strongly enough by statisticians or editors

ment. Standardisation was in doubt in 15 out of 38 clinical trials that I reviewed from the *Lancet* (July to December 1977).

In *Measurement in Medicine*[11] Oldham distinguished between qualitative and quantitative disagreement. The latter is disagreement on the intensity of the evidence—for example, in support of a diagnosis of multiple sclerosis—and not on the interpretation—for example, the presence or absence of a clinical sign. The figure shows that certain disagreements (shaded) have less serious implications than others in the diagnosis of multiple sclerosis by two neurologists,[3] and these instances of observer variation may be considered more leniently.

There are other solutions to between-observer variation. By randomising patients to the observers all of the different types of patients should be proportionately represented in the sample that is assessed by each observer. Each report should have an observer code or signature on it to identify which observer has assessed which patient. Subsequent observations on a particular patient must be made by the observer who recorded the patient's first result to avoid confounding of observer and treatment effects. I was told the story of the senior house officer who after having examined a patient compared his finding with the consultant's notes and was alarmed by the apparent deterioration. The consultant reviewed the case and pronounced an improvement. Beware between-observer variation. It may be necessary to defer the clinical trial until a better measurement scheme has been worked out or to appoint someone to do all the trial assessments.

(26) *In what way do the observations by clinician C differ from the others?*

—systematic error by observer C

Circum-corneal hyperaemia (scored 0,1,2,3,4) by four ophthalmologists												
Ophthalmologist	Patient											
	1	2	3	4	5	6	7	8	9	10	11	12
A	3	2	2	2	2	2	1	2	2	1	1	2
B	3	3	2	2	3	2	2	2	2	2	2	2
C	4	4	3	3	4	4	2	3	3	3	3	4
D	3	3	1	2	2	2	1	3	3	1	2	2

COMMENT

Circum-corneal hyperaemia (only for the lower half, avoiding the area of the cataract incision) was defined as: 0, normal; 1, conjunctival oedema; 2, conjunctival oedema+small venous engorgement; 3, conjunctival oedema+large venous engorgement; 4, unable to define underlying sclera.

Observer C systematically scored patients higher for circum-corneal hyperaemia than the other ophthalmologists did. Observer B scores in the middle of the range.

(27) *Comment on the assessment of iris hyperaemia by the four ophthalmologists.*

—**poor agreement**

—**carelessness (code 9)**

Ophthalmologist	Patient											
	1	2	3	4	5	6	7	8	9	10	11	12
A	1	0	0	0	0	3	1	2	0	0	0	1
B	1	0	1	4	1	1	1	1	4	1	0	1
C	4	0	0	0	0	4	0	4	9	0	0	0
D	3	3	1	1	2	2	1	2	2	1	2	2

Iris hyperaemia (scored 0,1,2,3,4) by four ophthalmologists

COMMENT

Iris hyperaemia was coded as follows: 0, nil; 1, proximity of iridectomies only—that is, less than 90°; 2, at least 90° and less than 180°; 3, at least 180° and less than 270°; 4, all quadrants.

The ophthalmologists vary unacceptably in their scoring of iris hyperaemia. Observer C uses only the extremes of the scale and introduces a spurious code—9—which has not been defined; observer D avoids the extreme codes. There is no patient on whom there is total agreement, and only three for whom the difference between the highest and lowest score is one. Observer variability is too large for this assessment to be of value in a clinical trial.

(28) *Observer variation in the clinical assessment of stroke was studied by Garraway et al.[4] Twelve patients were examined by consultants A, B, C, and D. The order of examination (figure) was balanced with respect to carry-over. Explain what a carry-over effect due to consultant A in the assessment of mental function means.*

—**consultant A leaves patients more (or less) able to answer the mental function questions than he found them**

Examination	Patient											
	1	2	3	4	5	6	7	8	9	10	11	12
1	A	B	C	D	A	B	C	D	A	B	C	D
2	B	A	D	C	C	D	A	B	D	C	B	A
3	C	D	A	B	D	C	B	A	B	A	D	C
4	D	C	B	A	B	A	D	C	C	D	A	B

COMMENT

The design selected by Garraway *et al*[4] was balanced for order of examination because patients might tire in an afternoon during which they had been examined four times. It was also balanced for carry-over from one examiner to the next, so that consultant A was followed equally often by consultants B, C, and D. Garraway *et al* found that whoever examined after consultant A scored mental function highly. An explanation was sought. It transpired that consultant A, a kindly man, put patients at their ease by telling them the answers to the questions on which they had failed. The information was retained over the short interval to the next examination but did not affect later assessments.

A carry-over from consultant A occurs if consultant A leaves patients more receptive to examination—or less receptive—than he found them.

The figure under question 25 showing observer variation between two neurologists has been reproduced from J R Landis and G G Koch. The measurement of observer agreement for categorical data. *Biometrics* 1977;**33**:159-74, with permission of the Biometric Society.

References

1 Rose G, Barker DJP. Repeatability and validity. *Epidemiology for the uninitiated*. London: British Medical Association, 1979.
2 Smyllie HC, Blendis LM, Armitage P. Observer disagreement in physical signs of the respiratory system. *Lancet* 1965;ii:412-3.
3 Landis JR, Koch GG. The measurement of observer agreement for categorical data. *Biometrics* 1977;**33**:159-74.
4 Garraway WM, Akhtar AJ, Gore SM, Prescott RJ, Smith RG. Observer variation in the clinical assessment of stroke. *Age and Ageing* 1976;**5**:233-40.
5 Wilson ME, Williams NB, Baskett PJF, Bennett JA, Skene AM. Assessment of fitness for surgical procedures and the variability of anaesthetists' judgments. *Br Med J* 1980;**280**:509-12.
6 Cochrane AL, Garland LH. Observer error in the interpretation of chest films—appendix C (PD Oldham). *Lancet* 1952;ii:505-9.
7 Yorkston JJ, Gruzelier JH, Zaki SA, Hollander D, Pitcher DR, Sergeant HGS. Propranolol as an adjunct to the treatment of schizophrenia. *Lancet* 1977;ii:575-8.
8 Rigby MJ, Chesham I. A trial speech screening test for school entrants. *Br Med J* 1981;**282**:449-51.
9 O'Brien ET, O'Malley K. ABC of blood pressure measurement—the observer. *Br Med J* 1979;ii:775-6.
10 Lehane A, O'Brien ET, O'Malley K. Reporting of blood pressure data in medical journals. *Br Med J* 1980;**281**:1603-4.
11 Oldham PD. Variation of observers' judgements. *Measurement in medicine*. London: English Universities Press, 1968.

ASSESSING CLINICAL TRIALS—
DOUBLE-BLIND TRIALS

The masking of observer and patient so that neither can identify the assigned treatment is the ideal way of avoiding subtly biased measurement (by the observer) or reporting (by the patient) of treatment outcome. Occasionally, response to treatment is unequivocal (death versus survival) so that double-blind comparison of treatments is a nicety of design rather than essential. More often treatments—for example, traction for low back pain—are such that double-blind comparison is practically impossible, though ingenious and valiant attempts have been made to cloak the assignments. Investigators are advised to describe how masking has been achieved or to explain clearly why comparison of masked treatments is not feasible.

(29) *What is meant by saying that a clinical trial is (i) double-blind; (ii) single-blind?*

(i) neither the assessor nor the patient can identify the assigned treatment

(ii) the assessor does not know the assigned treatment

COMMENT

(i) A clinical trial is double-blind (or double-masked) when neither the assessor nor the patient can identify the assigned treatment. In the Medical Research Council multicentre trial of glucagon and aprotinin in acute pancreatitis[1] patients were randomised in the ratio 1:1:2 to the three treatments: active aprotinin and glucagon placebo; active glucagon and aprotinin placebo; glucagon placebo and aprotinin placebo. The matched placebos were supplied by pharmaceutical companies and all patients appeared to receive both drugs.

(ii) If the identity of the treatment is concealed only from the assessor then the trial is single-masked or single-blind. A comparison of cytotoxic drugs can seldom be double-masked because treatments, distinguished by their side effects or schedule of dosage, are apparent to both patient and doctor. White blood cell count and the results of a biopsy may nevertheless be reported unbiasedly because it is usually possible to ensure that neither the haematologist nor the pathologist is informed about the patient's treatment. The term "single-blind" has also been applied to trials in which only the patient is in the dark, although this is not nearly so important as the assessor being in the dark.

(30) *When is it important that a clinical trial is single or double-blind?*

—when knowing the assigned treatment risks bias on the part of the assessor (observing) or the patient (reporting/experiencing response)

—when response is measured and is not objective

COMMENT

When knowledge of the patient's treatment might introduce bias to the doctor's assessment of the response to treatment the trial should be at least single-blind. If, moreover, the patient's response to the treatment or his reporting of that response might be prejudiced by knowing which treatment he receives the clinical trial should be double-blind or double-masked.

Bias in the recording of date of death is unusual. Systematic error in the reporting of time to the development of metastasis is possible, however, if one treatment group is unwittingly followed up more regularly than the others or if the methods used to detect metastases vary between treatment groups.

Prejudging a particular treatment may lead to unconsciously biased reporting of the clinical history, blood pressure, cell counts, radiographic films, biochemical test results, and many other measurements. A professor of my acquaintance has said that his assistants are keener on his ideas than he is himself.

> Anticipation: "a positive result will please the boss"

Anticipation—"a positive result will delight the boss"—is one of the 13 mortal sins of clinical assessment.[2]

The Northwick Park trial of electroconvulsive treatment (ECT)[3] is an interesting example of double-blind comparison between real and simulated ECT. The treatment allocation was known only to the psychiatrist who administered the ECT and to the anaesthetist. Neither of these doctors helped to care for or assess the patients; moreover, the patients, who completed scales for the self-assessment of anxiety and depression, did not know to which treatment group they belonged. The preconceived notions that the patients may have had about the effectiveness of electroconvulsive treatment could therefore hardly bias their response.

(31) *What tell-tale signs can unmask treatments?*

—smell, taste, shape, colour

—frequency (bd or tid)

—conversation between doctor and patient

—side effects

COMMENT

The tell-tale signs[4][5] that can unmask treatments include their smell, taste, or texture. Phillips and co-workers[6] compared atenolol versus adrenaline eye drops and the two combined in the treatment of glaucoma. Although eye discomfort was negligible, an unusual taste distinguished the "active" drops from the saline drops. The authors were careful not to claim that the trial was double-masked. In the South Wales dextran trial[7] one anaesthetist was suspected of attempting to differentiate between the dextran and placebo solutions by shaking them.

Other clues are the shape or colour either of the drugs themselves or of their containers. Frequency of administration—for example, bd versus tid—or toxicity is sometimes sufficient to distinguish treatments. Moreover, in single-blind trials the patient may simply tell the radiographer, tonometrist, or registrar which treatment has been given.

Anderson *et al*[5] have questioned the rather loose way in which the term "double-blind" is often used in the reports of clinical trials, suggesting that authors state what steps were taken to ensure that the preparations were indistinguishable, and, moreover, test the effectiveness of these measures. In a double-blind trial to test whether beta-blockade affected surgical performance[8] seven surgeons each took a 40 mg tablet of oxprenolol or placebo one hour before four operating sessions. The order of tablets had been randomised so that each surgeon took a 40 mg tablet of oxprenolol before two sessions and a matched placebo tablet before the other two sessions. After completing each operating list the surgeons were asked: "Did you take a beta-blocker?" Out of 28 responses the surgeons were wrong 17 times and correct 11 times and so were surprisingly unaware of whether they had taken oxprenolol or placebo.

Of course, blind comparison of treatments is not always possible. In a trial that compared the wound infection rate after abdominal operation[9] patients were randomly allocated to (*a*) an untreated control group, (*b*) a group receiving preoperative lincomycin and tobramycin, or (*c*) a group that received a local infusion of povidone-iodine. A survey of clinical trials published in the *Lancet* from July to December 1977 indicated that about half the trials that could have been double-blind were so. Investigators may have been reluctant to explain why masking was not feasible. Such explanation should be encouraged and ridiculous comments avoided—such as, "Patients were instructed to swallow the tablets without tasting them as taste could have interfered with the double-blind nature of the trial."

Double blind ?

Smell

Taste

Shape

Colour

Conversation between patient and doctor

Frequency

b d

t i d

Side effects

(32) *Guttae atenolol and guttae adrenaline are compared in a double-blind randomised cross-over trial. Elderly patients with glaucoma attend hospital for all-day tonometry on two study days. The contents of the bottle labelled "Patient 3, Day 1" have evaporated. Patient 3 is waiting. What should the tonometrist do?*

—use the assignment for patient 3, day 2

COMMENT

The tonometrist solved the problem neatly. She rejected the first five solutions for the reasons shown and settled for the sixth.

Solution 1 Send the patient home—was rejected because a return visit would impose an unnecessary burden on an elderly patient. Moreover, the trial design assumed that groups of four patients would attend together.

Double-masked randomised controlled trial in ophthalmology

Problem: the contents of the bottle labelled "Patient 3, Day 1" have evaporated

Solution: ?

Solution 2 Use the assignment for "patient 4, day 1"—was unacceptable because that patient had also come to hospital.

Solution 3 Withdraw patient 3—was rejected because reduction in patient numbers should be avoided and patient 3 would have made a wasted journey.

Solution 4 Replace the contents of the bottle—was impossible because the tonometrist did not know what the contents had been.

Solution 5 Statistician breaks the randomisation code to enable the pharmacy to replace the eye-drops—seems to be acceptable provided that the treatment code is not revealed to the tonometrist. But a further constraint is that ocular tension shows diurnal variation and a strict time schedule was imposed on the study. Unless the replacement could be made quickly this solution would also be inadequate.

Solution 6 Use the assignment for "patient 3, day 2"—was adopted. The patient was neither sent away nor kept waiting; the time schedule for the trial was adhered to; the tonometrist and the patient remained masked. The statistician was contacted before the patient's second visit and replacement drops obtained from the pharmacy. The balance of the trial design was slightly perturbed but that was the statistician's problem.

The example is included as a reminder that the double-blind nature of a clinical trial may make for unusual experimental difficulties. It is important to have an arrangement whereby the treatment code may be broken if a patient is withdrawn from the trial and subsequent care depends upon which trial treatment the patient was assigned to. It is often possible to specify an emergency treatment that may be used on any patient in need *without* breaking the code; and this should be arranged, if possible. In a long-term clinical study, if it is important that treatment allocation is not revealed to the trial doctors, a peer review group should be appointed with whom the statistician can discuss interim results and who will adjudicate for their colleagues on ethical issues. Only analyses of the trial as a whole (without reference to individual treatments) are presented to the participants in the trial.

References

[1] MRC Multi-centre Trial of Glucagon and Aprotinin. Death from acute pancreatitis. *Lancet* 1977;ii:632-5.
[2] Hart FD, Huskisson EW. Measurement in rheumatoid arthritis. *Lancet* 1972;i:28-30.

[3] Johnstone EC, Deakin JFW, Lawler P, *et al.* The Northwick Park electro-convulsive therapy trial. *Lancet* 1980;ii:1317-20.

[4] Hill LE, Nunn AJ, Fox W. Matching quality of agents employed in "double-blind" controlled clinical trials. *Lancet* 1976;i:352-6.

[5] Anderson TW, Ashley MJ, Clarke EA. Not so double-blind? *Br Med J* 1976;i:457-8.

[6] Phillips CI, Gore SM, Gunn PM. Atenolol versus adrenaline eye drops and an evaluation of these two combined. *Br J Ophthalmol* 1978;**62**:296-301.

[7] Davies TW. Dextran or heparin? *Lancet* 1978;ii:1315-6.

[8] Foster GE, Makin C, Evans DF, Hardcastle JW. Does β-blockade affect surgical performance? A double blind trial of oxprenolol. *Br J Surg* 1980;**67**:609-12.

[9] Galland RB, Saunders JH, Mosley JG, Darrell JH. Prevention of wound infection in abdominal operations by preoperative antibiotics or povidone-iodine. *Lancet* 1977;ii:1043-5.

ASSESSING CLINICAL TRIALS—
TRIAL DISCIPLINE

Several questions about trial discipline are raised here that must be answered satisfactorily before the clinical study begins. It is important to decide whether a fixed-dose or a variable-dose regimen is appropriate—they are different treatments—to realise that including a vehicle treatment (or placebo) may be unethical and is not a necessary part of clinical trial methodology. Consideration should be given to ways of enhancing or monitoring compliance with treatment and follow-up of patients. The routine for examining patients should be carefully determined and, when appropriate, a time table drawn up. Ocular tension, for example, shows diurnal variation and so should be measured at fixed times by one tonometrist. Blood pressure should also be recorded under standard conditions—for example, sitting blood pressure after two minutes' sitting and specified cut-off for diastolic pressure.

Fixed or variable dose

(33) *Investigators are tempted to compare fixed-dose regimens merely to facilitate double-blind comparison of treatments. When should this temptation be resisted?*

—when there is considerable variation between patients in the dosage required to produce a therapeutic effect

—to avoid getting answers to clinically trivial questions

COMMENT

This temptation should be resisted when a considerable variation in the dosage between patients is required to produce a pharmacological effect. For example, in diabetes the dose is tailored to the patient's need, and so should it be also in a clinical trial; otherwise, as Ritter[1] suggests, we risk getting "highly reliable answers to inherently trivial questions." For practical purposes in clinical trials comparisons should be made between treatments that are optimally prescribed.[2] Only then is the relevant clinical problem tackled. It will not do to alter the prescription of one drug to bring it in line with another to force double-blind comparison if by modifying the regimen you interfere with the drug's effectiveness. In such circumstances double-blind comparison must be abandoned, and clinical importance takes priority. Arrange for an independent blind assessment when the differences between treatments cannot realistically be concealed from the patient. Fixed regimen has been criticised in electroconvulsive treatment[3] and in the use of beta-blocking drugs[1]: investigators valued double-blind comparison too highly, perhaps with the loss of therapeutic activity.

Placebo treatment

(34) *When is the inclusion in a clinical trial of a placebo treatment justified?*

—when there is no recognised proved management for the disease, and in addition a non-specific psychological effect is suspected or observer bias is likely

COMMENT

The pragmatic view of a clinical trial is that the control arm should be an accepted treatment for the disease in question. Only then do the results of the trial answer the relevant clinical question: "Does the new treatment improve on a standard method?" The explanation that a new drug is better than no treatment may interest drug regulatory authorities but has no practical implication for the treatment of patients.[4]

To include an untreated group or a sham or inactive treatment group, or both, in trials that ask a practical question about how to treat—that is, in pragmatic trials—is warranted only if there is no recognised proved management for the disease. If so, and a non-specific psychological or psychophysiological effect is suspected or observer bias is likely, a group treated with placebo should be included as well as or instead of untreated patients. Schwartz *et al*[5] referred to an example that showed how readily a doctor's expectation was translated into "fact." An astonishing response to a new drug was noted in a patient with asthma for whom other treatments had been tried without success. There was a consistently poor response when a placebo was substituted for the new drug. No one was more surprised than the doctor who, having written to congratulate the drug firm, was informed that they had supplied him only with placebo.

Deliberate denial of an effective treatment is wrong unless patients give fully informed consent to it and there is also ethical

"There is no justification for many of the placebo trials, apart from the speed with which the statisticians can be satisfied" WRONG

There is no justification for many of the placebo trials
Reason: there may be all the difference in the world between statistical significance and biological significance

approval (conditions which are rarely met). The accusation that the only justification for many of the placebo trials that are reported is the speed with which the statisticians can be satisfied is equally wrong!

Although much ingenuity is channelled into preparing sham inert treatments occasionally there is an unfortunate error, as when lactose powder—"a nutrient substrate eminently utilisable by large-bowel organisms"[6]—was chosen as a placebo in a trial to compare methods for reducing postoperative wound infection.

Order of examination

(35) *What is wrong with the procedure illustrated?*

—the same doctor first interviews the patient and then performs an endoscopy

—the second assessment may be biased by the information he has got from the interview

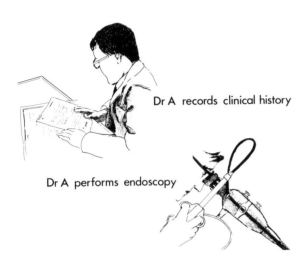

Dr A records clinical history

Dr A performs endoscopy

COMMENT

The same doctor first interviews the patient and then performs an endoscopy. The information about symptoms and the patient's perception of how successful treatment has been may thus prejudice the endoscopic findings. The doctor may see what he expects to see. A better arrangement is for one doctor to take the patient's history and a second doctor, who has not read these clinical notes, perform the endoscopy, so that the second assessment is independent of the first.

In a study[7] of symptoms in middle life special care was taken not to mention menopause in the first questionnaire, which asked about whether some 40 different symptoms had occurred. The covering letter said merely that the study was concerned with the health problems of men and women of working age. The second questionnaire, sent about eight weeks later, investigated family, social, and gynaecological matters and treatment and so contained material that might have biased responses to the first questionnaire if the two had not been separated. Bias was the eighth of 13 mortal sins of clinical assessment.[8]

Two other faults are change of assessor and change in the time of assessment. The first, and usually also the second, should be determined in the list of the trial procedures. In the Northwick Park trial of electroconvulsive treatment (ECT)[9] treatments were given on Tuesdays and Fridays. Patients who began their course of ECT on a Tuesday were rated on five consecutive Mondays, and those who began their course on a Friday were rated on five consecutive Thursdays. In a trial on essential hypertension[10] patients were examined at a fixed time of day and instructed to take their tablets at the same time each day. In such studies blood pressure should be measured by the same observer throughout and the procedure carefully defined.

Compliance

(36) *What steps can be taken to enhance treatment compliance or to monitor it, or both?*

—simplify instructions

—use a calendar pack (for example, oral contraceptives)

—practice (for example, how to use inhalers)

—use a diary card as a reminder

—return unused drugs

—observe (spectacles worn?)

—analyse blood or urine samples (spot checks)

COMMENT

Simplifying the regimen, provided that this is consistent with pharmacological activity, minimises errors of comprehension and errors of memory. Prescribing medication once daily or timing doses to correspond with mealtimes or other regular activities helps[11]; training patients before discharging them how to use their medicines—for example, inhalers—providing labels that are easy to read and convenient packaging—for example, calendar packs—and providing a diary card make it simpler for the patient to adhere to the prescribed routine. Unpleasant taste or smell may inhibit compliance. Liquid and tablet De-Nol were compared[12] for efficacy and acceptability in the treatment of duodenal ulcer.

In an explanatory clinical trial, which is devised to answer a question about the therapeutic activity of a particular regimen,

Diary card			
Day	Time	Dose	Check
Mon (18·5·81)	8am	2 tablets	✓
	6pm	1 tablet	✓
Tues (19·5·81)	8am	2 tablets	✓
	6pm	1 tablet	
"	"	"	
Sun (24·5·81)	8am	2 tablets	
	6pm	1 tablet	

compliance with that regimen is important and should be checked. A different question is whether the regimen is efficient in practice, when inevitably patients vary in compliance. This second pragmatic study does not differentiate at analysis between those patients who comply strictly and those who lapse, though it still may be important to measure the degree of compliance and observe the disease and other characteristics of patients who fail to follow instructions.

Treatment compliance may be monitored by asking patients to bring their medicines with them for inspection when they attend the clinic, and by asking them to return all unused trial drugs. Patients may easily dispose of an incriminating surplus if they have a mind to, of course. But the results of even such a naive check may be startlingly informative—for instance, the patient who knows that the doctor has changed the tablets because they don't float when they are flushed down the lavatory. Peckham *et al*[13] found that 17% of children who had been prescribed and needed spectacles were not wearing them when they attended for an eye examination. The true proportion of non-users is likely to be even higher.

A more reliable monitor is the analysis of blood or urine samples. Elwood and Sweetnam[14] compared aspirin versus placebo in preventing secondary mortality after myocardial infarction. Additional home visits were made without warning and a urine sample requested to measure salicylate. The results suggested that the compliance rate was at least 72% (due consideration was given to false-positive and false-negative rates).

Lionel and Herxheimer have produced a check-list for assessing reports of therapeutic trials[15] in which they include monitoring of compliance.

(37) *What can be done to minimise the loss to follow-up of patients in a clinical trial?*

—careful definition of the study population in the first instance

—issue reminders when appointments are missed

—avoid unnecessarily lengthy or complicated forms

—maintain enthusiasm for the trial

COMMENT

The proportion of studies in which patients are lost to follow-up or withdrawn in retrospect is high. In 20 out of 38 clinical trials reported in the *Lancet* from July to December 1977 patients were withdrawn or excluded because follow-up had lapsed. Loss to follow-up and withdrawal of patients from a clinical trial may be minimised by (*a*) a careful check before registration on the eligibility of the patient to enter the trial; (*b*) restriction of the study population (and hence also restriction of the implications of the trial) to patients for whom examinations for the clinical trial are not a serious imposition either domestically or physically; (*c*) the diligent issue of reminders when

appointments are missed. It is also the responsibility of the trial co-ordinator to know as early as possible about lapses in the trial procedures and to report these at meetings of trial participants so that corrections may be made. Nothing is more destructive of enthusiastic collaboration than for doctors to be faced with unnecessarily lengthy or complicated recording forms, which are time consuming to complete. Simplified trial procedures that are discussed and agreed before the trial starts and verified in pilot studies do much to ensure co-operation and follow-up. In multicentre trials visits to the centres by the trial co-ordinator are more effective than sending impersonal progress reports.

References

1 Ritter JM. Placebo-controlled, double-blind clinical trials can impede medical progress. *Lancet* 1980;i:1126-7.
2 Schwartz D, Flamant R, Lellouch J. Problem formulation. *Clinical trials* London: Academic Press, 1980.
3 Gordon D. The Northwick Park ECT trial. *Lancet* 1981;i:284.
4 Anonymous. Controlled trials: planned deception? *Lancet* 1979;i:534-5.
5 Schwartz D, Flamant R, Lellouch J. The placebo effect. *Clinical trials* London: Academic Press, 1980.
6 Whitfield PJ. Treating preinfected wounds. *Br Med J* 1969;iv:428.
7 Bungay GT, Vessey MP, McPherson CK. Study of symptoms in middle life with special reference to the menopause. *Br Med J* 1980;281:181-3.
8 Hart FD, Huskisson EW. Measurement in rheumatoid arthritis. *Lancet* 1972;i:28-30.
9 Johnstone EC, Deakin JFW, Lawler P, *et al.* The Northwick Park ECT trial. *Lancet* 1980;ii:1317-20.
10 Pearson RM, Bulpitt CJ, Havard CWH. Biochemical and haematological changes induced by tienilic acid combined with propranolol in essential hypertension. *Lancet* 1979;i:697-9.
11 Norell SE. Improving medication compliance: a randomised clinical trial. *Br Med J* 1979;ii:1031-3.
12 Hamilton I, Axon ATR. Controlled trial comparing De-Nol tablets with De-Nol liquid in treatment of duodenal ulcer. *Br Med J* 1981;282:362
13 Peckham CS, Gardiner PA, Tibbenham A. Vision screening of adolescents and their use of glasses. *Br Med J* 1979;i:1111-3.
14 Elwood PC, Sweetnam PM. Aspirin and secondary mortality after myocardial infarction. *Lancet* 1979;ii:1313-5.
15 Lionel NDW, Herxheimer A. Assessing reports of therapeutic trials. *Br Med J* 1970;iii:637-40.

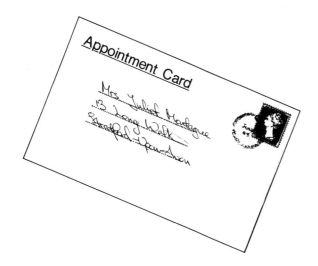

ASSESSING CLINICAL TRIALS—
RECORD SHEETS

The attempt to record too much information leads to carelessness and lack of enthusiasm by the trial participants. Beware of this pitfall, particularly in long-term or multicentre trials. Having separate record sheets for each assessment—interview, physical examination, chest radiography—and for each visit helps to avoid observer bias. Note that it is important to code missing values—for example, tumour size unknown=99—to avoid confusion between a blank (unknown or not recorded?) and zero (no measurable mass). Precoding—male=1, female=2—makes computer processing easy; avoid code 0.

(38) *Neat layout is important. Compare records A and B.*

—**record B is better**

—**answers are precoded numerically on record B**

—**failure to record (blank) and no available information (missing-value code) cannot easily be distinguished in record A**

—**for record B only there is a simple correspondence between the coding sheet and the columns of a computer record**

COMMENT

Both records have a neat and orderly layout. In record A the clinical case history is noted in the left-hand column and the treatment and the outcome of disease are recorded on the right. Record B, like record A, is a single sheet on which the clinical notes are made before the decision about the treatment and survival status of the patient are entered. This order corresponds with the natural sequence of events.

The advantage that record B has over record A is that answers are precoded numerically to facilitate data processing; missing-value codes are assigned so that whoever checks the record may distinguish, for most items, between failure to record (blank) and no available information (missing-value code). It is much more difficult to transfer information correctly from record A

A

Name
Hospital number
Date of birth

Age	
Menstrual status	Primary treatment
premenopause	simple mastectomy
menopause	radiotherapy
postmenopause	radical mastectomy
unknown	other
Side	Site of first metastasis
	visceral
Tumour size	bone
	other breast
Fixation to skin	
partial	Date of primary treatment
complete	
	Date of first metastasis
Ulceration	
	Date of death
Peau d'orange	
tumour area	Cause of death
breast	
Satellite nodules skin	Status at 1980 anniversary
Invasive to skin wide of breast	
	Length of survival
Deep fixation	
fascia	
muscle	
chest wall	
Homolateral axillary nodes	
mobile	
matted	
Other nodes	
Lymphoedema	
Metastasis at presentation	
skin	
distant	
International stage	

B

Name

Hospital number
Date of birth

Age in completed years				
Menstrual status	premenopause = 1	menopause = 2	postmenopause = 3	15
	not known = 9			
Side	left = 1	right = 2	bilateral = 3	16
Tumour size (cms)	not known = 99			
Fixation to skin	nil = 1	partial = 2	complete = 3	19
Ulceration				20
Peau d'orange - tumour area				21
breast				22
Satellite nodules skin				23
Invasive skin wide of breast	no = 1	yes = 2		24
Deep fixation - fascia				25
muscle				26
chest wall				27
Homolateral axillary nodes	not involved = 1	mobile = 2	matted = 3	28
Other nodes				29
Lymphoedema	no = 1	yes = 2		30
Metastasis at presentation - skin				31
distant				32
International stage	not known = 9			33
Primary treatment				
simple mastectomy	no = 1	yes = 2		34
radiotherapy	no = 1	yes = 2		35
radical mastectomy	no = 1	yes = 2		36
other	no = 1	yes = 2		37
Site of first metastasis				
visceral	no = 1	yes = 2		38
bone	no = 1	yes = 2		39
other breast	no = 1	yes = 2		40
Date of first treatment	not known = 0			
Date of first metastasis	not known = 0			
Date of death	not known = 0			
Cause of death	breast cancer = 1	other causes = 2	alive = 3	59
Status at 1980 anniversary	alive = 1	lost to follow up = 2	dead = 3	60
Survival in completed years				

to a computer file because doctors are left to devise their own coding conventions (a tick, an X, YES), and there is not a simple correspondence between the coding sheet and the columns of a computer record.

(39) *What checks should be made at the hospital before records are sent to the statistician?*

—check completeness and legibility

—check that all codes are valid

—check that there are no gross errors (date of mastectomy 23-05-67, date of death 18-08-63)

—keep a record of posting

COMMENT

Before records are sent to the statistician a check should be made that every item has a valid code, that the forms are easily legible, and that there are no gross errors—such as date of death preceding date of treatment. A computer program will, of course, be written to detect logical errors, slips in coding, and key punching mistakes. Incorrect records are then referred back to the hospital for checking. Verification is important but time-consuming, and to keep it to a minimum make the appropriate checks before the data are sent for processing.

It is wise for the hospital to keep a log of the forms (on-study form; annual follow-up 1, 2, 3, 4; end of study form) that they have posted and for the data-processing staff also to register that they have received the coding sheets by keeping a similar log.

(40) *What means is there of ensuring that both the hospital and the statistician hold copies of the patient record sheets?*

—photocopy records

COMMENT

The simplest means of ensuring that both the hospital and the statistician hold copies of the patient record sheets is to photocopy the record. If record sheets are colour-coded—for example, on-study form, white; follow-up form, blue; end of

Photocopy machine

Pencil   Legibility   Coloured form

study form, yellow—it may be necessary to maintain the colour code in the photocopies also. The quality of a photocopy may be poor if a pencil or blue ink has been used to complete the original record sheet and the copy and the original have to be compared before despatch.

(41) *Always find out from those who complete the form if there are difficulties using it. What is wrong with the layout of this form for recording intraocular pressure?*

—the columns for right and left eye have been inter-changed

—the patient's right eye is on the tonometrist's left as she faces the patient; so it should be also on the form

Form for recording intraocular pressure

Patient's hospital number _____		
Patient's study number _____		
Date of examination _____		

Time (hours)	Left eye	Right eye
09·00		
11·00		
13·00		
15·00		
17·00		

COMMENT

I asked the chief tonometrist at the Princess Alexandra Eye Pavilion in Edinburgh to approve this form for recording intraocular pressure before I had it duplicated. She told me that it would not do. I wondered why—it was simple, neat, and unambiguous. Or was it? The patient's right eye is, of course, on the tonometrist's left as she faces the patient and ought to be so on the form also. Therefore the form should be redesigned as shown.

Time (hours)	Right eye	Left eye
09.00		
11.00		

If experience is the sum of one's errors then I, for one, have learned a vast amount, and one of the most valuable lessons is always to check out form design with the person who will do the recording and, for all but the simplest forms, to pilot them before the trial proper begins.[1] Useful pointers on form design have been given by Wright and Haybittle.[2]

References

[1] Cancer Research Campaign Working Party. Trials and tribulations: thoughts on the organisation of multicentre clinical studies. *Br Med J* 1980;**281**:918-20.
[2] Wright P, Haybittle J. Design of forms for clinical trials. *Br Med J* 1979;ii:529-2, 650-1.

ASSESSING CLINICAL TRIALS—
PROTOCOL AND MONITORING

The question of whether a patient is eligible for a clinical trial is resolved by the doctor checking through the list of entrance requirements to be met—diagnostic tests, clinical state, previous treatment, other disease. The doctor should also ensure that there is no reason specifically to exclude the patient because of treatment preference, contraindications, or possibly biased response (see question 42). A good practice is to keep a log of all patients who satisfy the trial diagnosis, and against each name register either clinical trial number or the entrance requirement or exclusion clause that debarred the individual patient. In this way the investigators define the class of patients about whose treatment inferences will be made from the trial results and also estimate the proportion of patients that this class represents of all the patients who satisfy the diagnostic criteria.

As a general rule entrance criteria should be less restrictive when the aim is to compare treatment policies and so reach a practical decision about how to treat than if the trial has an explanatory purpose, such as discovering how treatments work. A good discussion on this point is given by Mosteller et al.[1] Moreover, in practice the entrance requirements will usually be tailored to ensure that patients are followed up completely and considerately. Thus there may be an age barrier, or patients may be excluded because they have other disease, because their life expectancy is shorter than the study period (except, of course, when survival is the endpoint of the trial), because they are not mobile, or because their families cannot cope adequately. The rules should be simply defined, agreed by the participating doctors and interpreted uniformly by them. Investigators should recognise that limiting the study population also limits the generality of their findings.

Besides defining the entrance criteria the trial protocol gives details of design, randomisation, checks that will be made on how the study is being conducted, and information about how the data will be handled. But the protocol is important for another—sometimes forgotten—reason. It sets down the comparisons between treatments that the investigation has been designed to make, thereby setting them apart form hypotheses that are suggested after the trial results are known. The analysis should be thought through when the design of the clinical trial is being considered. This outline analysis is then written into the protocol and computer programs prepared in advance, as necessary.

Specific exclusions

(42) *Describe three types of patients who should be specifically excluded from randomised comparison of treatments.*

—patients for whom a trial treatment is contraindicated

—patients whose response to particular treatments may be biased

—patients for whom the doctor has a definite treatment preference

COMMENT

Patients for whom one of the trial treatments is contraindicated differ in respect of that contraindication—and perhaps also in other respects related to outcome—from patients who may receive any one of the rival treatments without harm. Therefore patients for whom a trial treatment is contraindicated should be specifically excluded. Treatment with beta-blockers, for example, is not advised for patients with asthma; such patients were ineligible for the trial in which Wilcox et al[2] compared propranolol, atenolol, and placebo in the immediate treatment of myocardial infarction. Also ineligible, but for a different reason, were patients who were already taking a beta-blocker. In this case the specific exclusion was necessary because synergism (or antagonism) of drugs could not be ruled out. Patients whose response to particular treatments may be biased should be excluded. A second example comes from a study in neuropsychology about which I was consulted. It compared "reality orientation schemes" for geriatric patients. In two of the schemes patients were instructed how to make things. Group instruction was practicable only if patients could hear well. Elderly patients who were deaf were therefore excluded because their response to two of the treatments would be impaired. As a consequence the conclusions applied also only to patients who had an adequate level of hearing. Thirdly, exclude any patient for whom the doctor has a definite treatment preference. As described in the introduction a log should be kept of patients who are specifically excluded with the reason for their ineligibility.

	Entrance criteria
Example	Double-blind randomised controlled trial to compare topical antiglaucoma agents, one of which is a beta-blocker
Entrance criteria	Previously untreated patients who have simple open-angle glaucoma or ocular hypertension [unilateral or bilateral]
	Patients must be well enough to attend hospital for all day tonometry on four study days at intervals of one week
Specific exclusions	Specifically exclude patients with cardiovascular disease
	Specifically exclude patients who are being treated with a systemic beta-blocker
	Specifically exclude patients for whom the ophthalmologist has a definite treatment preference

Protocol

(43) *An orderly presentation of the details of the design, organisation, and outline analysis for a clinical trial is shown below. Why is full documentation important?*

—the protocol is a record not only of decisions made but also of the reasoning or calculation that led to those decisions

—trial procedures should be fully described

—documentation should be sufficiently detailed for the statistician to pick up quickly the threads of the study

COMMENT

Careful documentation is important because the report on a clinical trial is usually written months or years after the first patient is entered. The protocol stands as a record for the authors—of the decisions made and also of the reasoning or calculation that led to those decisions. The protocol will, of course, be incomplete as a reference unless any modifications that were made to the trial procedure during accrual or follow-up are described in an appendix, noting the date, nature of, and reason for changing the procedure.

The second reason for full documentation is the inevitability that clinical investigators will change. New participants must become familiar with the trial procedures, which are described in the protocol. Lastly, documentation should be sufficiently detailed for the statistician quickly to pick up the threads of the study when the time comes for interim or final analysis. Otherwise, important comparisons may be overlooked or a less sensitive analysis reported because the critical features of the study design have been forgotten.

Protocol

(1) Title, list of centres entering patients, job description of trial organisers, date of trial starting
(2) Aim of investigation
(3) Ethical consideration, pilot studies
(4) Entrance criteria
(5) Criteria for withdrawal or exclusion
(6) Response variables (and priority if there is more than one measure of response)
(7) Covariates, recording sheets as appendix
(8) Trial organisation
   treatment assignment (locally or centrally, sealed envelopes. . .), treatment details (fixed or variable dose, administration (qid)), observers, time of visits, timing of assessments, order of assessments
(9) Design
   historical data (referenced), size of clinically important difference and power requirements, fixed or sequential design, size of clinical trial (calculation as appendix), between- or within-patient study, method of randomisation (randomisation list is held in camera)
(10) Plan of analysis
   treatment comparisons of interest, assumptions about response distribution, handling of missing observations, withdrawal, exclusions, loss to follow-up, reversed treatments, frequency of interim analyses and their formality

JUSTIFY DECISIONS MADE

Indeed the protocol should be written clearly enough for the trial to be repeated elsewhere and analysed in a similar fashion. An aide-memoire for preparing clinical trial protocols is useful.[3]

Checks on trial conduct

(44) *Checks on trial conduct are particularly important in long-term studies. What type of check should be made, and why?*

For ethical reasons:
—toxicity

—excess mortality from a particular cause

—important treatment difference

Unstable trial conditions:
—rate of patient entry

—rate of withdrawal

—change in distribution of baseline patient characteristics (age, tumour stage . . .)

—change over time in level of response to all treatments

—change in level of response to a particular treatment

COMMENT

Ethical considerations oblige the statistician to review periodically accumulating data from long-term studies for evidence of toxicity, excessive mortality from a particular cause (as in the University Group Diabetes Program[4]), or important treatment difference. To account properly for repeated significance testing the trial design should specify the number of such interim analyses and when they will be performed.

Most other checks are made to detect instability in the trial conditions. Thus a tailing off in the rate of patient accrual is often the first sign that investigators have lost enthusiasm for the trial and a progress report is urgently called for. A change in the rate of patient withdrawal from the study is a warning that entrance criteria have been relaxed to admit patients who would have been deemed unsuitable before or that there has been a systematic change in the assessment of how severe the side effects of treatment are. Other indications of a subtle alteration in the type of patient admitted to the study are change in the distribution of baseline patient characteristics—such as age at diagnosis, tumour stage, histology—or in the level of response to all treatments. Change in the overall level of response could also be accounted for by a drift in the measurement of response. A change in the level of response to a particular treatment is equally alarming. Possible explanations are a leak in the assignment scheme so that selection bias operates, a change in drug formulation (batch number, for example) or biased assessment because the observer is no longer blind to the assigned treatment.

The execution of a clinical trial is the most exacting phase for doctors; it should not be a period of quiescence for the statistician.

References

[1] Mosteller F, Gilbert JP, McPeek B. Reporting standards and research strategies for controlled trials. Agenda for the editor. *Controlled Clinical Trials* 1980;**1**:37-58.
[2] Wilcox RG, Roland JM, Banks DC, Hampton JR, Mitchell JRA. Randomised trial comparing propranolol with atenolol in immediate treatment of suspected myocardial infarction. *Br Med J* 1980;**280**:885-8.
[3] Clinical Trials Unit, London Hospital Medical College. Aide-memoire for preparing clinical trial protocols. *Br Med J* 1977;i:1323-4.
[4] Cornfield J. The University Group Diabetes Program: a further statistical analysis of mortality findings. *JAMA* 1971;**217**:1676-87.

ASSESSING CLINICAL TRIALS— RASH ADVENTURES

Eagerness to begin analysis may compromise the careful planning and execution of the trial if the important step of checking the data before analysis is omitted. No amount of statistical ingenuity can make bad data good. What is needed is first to prepare an account of the numbers of patients lost to follow-up or withdrawn from the trial, giving the reasons for withdrawal and evaluating potential bias; secondly, to check that the observations are sensible—within range, for example—orderly, and consistent for a given patient; and thirdly, to compare baseline characteristics between randomised groups to verify that the patients in these groups are initially similar or to be aware of chance differences that should be taken into account at analysis.

Patient withdrawal

(45) *What information should be reported about patients who are withdrawn from a clinical trial or excluded retrospectively?*

—numbers of patients withdrawn from each treatment group

—reasons for withdrawal

—potential bias if these patients are not included at analysis

COMMENT

Patients are withdrawn from clinical trials or excluded retrospectively for a variety of reasons. These include the patient's refusal to continue in the study, lapsed attendance, loss to follow-up because of moving from the health authority, side effects or toxicity, intercurrent disease or death, eventual discovery that the patient does not meet the entrance criteria, treatment reversal whereby the patient received a treatment other than the randomised assignment, poor compliance, other protocol deviation such as dose limitation or intensification in response to the patient's clinical status. Therefore, besides reporting the actual numbers of patients withdrawn from each treatment group, trial investigators should in each case give the reason for withdrawal and the implications for analysis. Thus Wilcox et al[1] reported that 44 (33%) of 132 patients who were randomised to propranolol, 51 (40%) out of 127 on atenolol, and 40 (31%) out of 129 on placebo were withdrawn during the first six weeks after immediate treatment of suspected myocardial infarction. Although the numbers of withdrawals were similar for all the treatments, the reasons for withdrawal were very different. Forty-nine (52%) of the 95 patients withdrawn after treatment with beta-blockers compared with only five (13%) out of 40 placebo withdrawals were accounted for by hypotension or bradycardia. Trial results can be seriously biased by ignoring the outcome for patients who have suffered side effects, refused co-operation, shown poor compliance or in whom it has been necessary to modify the trial regimen. Most often the correct

analysis, as reported by Wilcox et al, is between groups of patients as randomised not as treated. (This is especially important in the case of possibly deliberate treatment reversal.) The rationale is for a pragmatic comparison on the basis of intention to treat—that is, between treatment policies.

When the trial is being designed investigators should list

> Follow up patients who have been withdrawn in exactly the same manner as patients who continue on treatment

possible reasons for patient withdrawal, assess how best to analyse the results from such patients to avoid bias, and write into the trial protocol the methods of analysis which will be required.

A good general principle is to follow up patients who have been withdrawn in exactly the same manner as patients who continue on treatment, provided that this is consistent with the patient's wishes. Patients who default often differ in outcome and prognosis from patients who comply. Treatment difference may be exaggerated, diminished, or reversed by thoughtless exclusion of relevant cases.

(46) *Assess the bias associated with patient withdrawal in the following examples:*

(*a*) In a prospective controlled trial of hyperbaric oxygen as an adjuvant in radiotherapy of head and neck cancer,[2] 151 patients were randomly allocated to treatment in air and 143 to treatment in hyperbaric oxygen. The endpoints were survival and disease-free interval. Eighteen patients allocated to hyperbaric oxygen could not be treated in the chamber because of claustrophobia or convulsions during the first compression. These 18 patients were excluded from the hyperbaric oxygen group and their results reported separately.

(*b*) Thirty-seven men with seronegative spondyloarthritis took part in a randomised controlled cross-over study that compared immune reactions stimulated by levamisole and placebo during each 12-week treatment phase.[3] Serious side effects led to withdrawal of the active drug in nine patients. Clinical response was compared in the remaining 28 patients.

(a) exclusion of the 18 patients makes a pragmatic comparison between treatment policies invalid;

the question of whether radiotherapy in hyperbaric oxygen is superior to radiotherapy in air in respect of patients who could have received either is probably answered by the authors' analysis

(b) toxicity is a severe indictment of any treatment

COMMENT

(a) Henk et al[2] reasoned that claustrophobia and oxygen toxicity were unlikely to be associated with the prognosis in malignant disease or to have any relation to the outcome of radiotherapy. They therefore excluded the 18 patients who could not be treated in the hyperbaric oxygen chamber from their main analysis, but took the precaution of reporting also the combined analysis. The two methods relate to different questions, the first to an explanatory purpose, the second to a pragmatic one.

Exclusion of the 18 patients makes a pragmatic comparison between treatment policies invalid; the trial results as first analysed do not represent a comparison between practicable treatments because there will always be head and neck cancer patients who suffer claustrophobia or oxygen toxicity for whom some (lesser?) treatment must be devised. The second analysis unbiasedly estimates the overall effect of the policy: treat in hyperbaric oxygen whenever possible and in air otherwise.

The question of whether radiotherapy in hyperbaric oxygen is superior to radiotherapy in air in respect of patients who could have received either is explanatory in nature. It is best answered by excluding from the trial before randomisation patients who have a history of claustrophobia or oxygen toxicity (because treatment in hyperbaric oxygen is contraindicated). If in practice preselection was difficult then the authors have, in their primary analysis, made the best answer they could to the explanatory question—an answer that is unbiased if the reasoning of the authors is correct.

(b) Toxicity is a severe indictment of any treatment, as Goebel et al[3] recognised when they reported on levamisole-induced immunostimulation in spondyloarthritis. Benefit in 28 patients was bought at the price of serious side effects in nine others. Until a method can be found of averting these side effects, which necessitated immediate withdrawal of the active drug in 25% of patients, immunostimulation by levamisole is a "two-edged sword."

Data inspection

(47) *The table gives a 10-point check-list for data inspection. What errors do you detect in the record shown (figure)?*

Data inspection: check-list

(1) Patient eligibility.
(2) Treatment assignment against randomisation list and order of trial numbers against entry dates (number 12: 10/3/80, number 13: 27/2/80).
(3) Completeness (blanks?) and correct sequence (1,2,?,4,5) of records for individual patients; serial order of patients in the trial as a whole (unallocated trial numbers?); observer code—standard per patient?
(4) Inadmissible codes: male = 1, female = 2, code 8 is undefined.
(5) Sensible range for every variable. I have encountered breast tumour 42 cm; age 3 years as the age when a patient started smoking; ocular tension 9 mm Hg in treated simple open-angle glaucoma. All are outside the usual range. All were queried—the first two were confirmed but the last, ocular tension, should have read 19 mm Hg. It did so on the original record of which I held an imperfect photocopy.
(6) Legibility.
(7) Accuracy of observations: be suspicious if some observations are recorded more accurately than others (different assessor, different instrument, carelessness?)—for example 1·64, 2·7, 1½, 2.
(8) Dates: 29 02 78 is in error because 1978 was not a leap year.

(9) Sequence of events: date of birth precedes date of mastectomy; date of metastasis is not later than date of death.
(10) Internal consistency: if tumour size is more than 5 cm then international stage is at least stage 3 breast cancer; a 60-year-old man is an unlikely patient in a hospital for sick children.

Field				Code/Value
Name				
Hospital number				1 0 0 7 5 6
Date of birth				3 1 0 4 2 0
Age in completed years				3 6
Menstrual status	premenopause = 1 not known = 9	menopause = 2	postmenopause = 3	15 [1]
Side	left = 1	right = 2	bilateral = 3	16 [2]
Tumour size (cms)	not known = 99			[4]
Fixation to skin	nil = 1	partial = 2	complete = 3	19 [illegible]
Ulceration				20 [2]
Peau d'orange - tumour area				21 [1]
breast				22 [1]
Satellite nodules skin		no = 1	yes = 2	23 [1]
Invasive skin wide of breast				24 [1]
Deep fixation - fascia				25 [1]
muscle				26 [1]
chest wall				27 [1]
Homolateral axillary nodes	not involved = 1	mobile = 2	matted = 3	28 [2]
Other nodes				29 [1]
Lymphoedema		no = 1	yes = 2	30 [1]
Metastasis at presentation - skin				31 [1]
distant				32 [1]
International stage	not known = 9			33 [2]
Primary treatment				
simple mastectomy	no = 1	yes = 2		34
radiotherapy	no = 1	yes = 2		35
radical mastectomy	no = 1	yes = 2		36
other	no = 1	yes = 2		37
Site of first metastasis				
visceral	no = 1	yes = 2		38 [2]
bone	no = 1	yes = 2		39 [1]
other breast	no = 1	yes = 2		40 [2]
Date of first treatment	not known = 0			2 9 1 1 6 6
Date of first metastasis	not known = 0			
Date of death	not known = 0			2 7 0 6 6 0
Cause of death	breast cancer = 1	other causes = 2	alive = 3	59 [1]
Status at 1980 anniversary	alive = 1	lost to follow up = 2	dead = 3	60 [1]
Survival in completed years				[3]

COMMENT

The errors contained in the record shown in the figure are as follows:

(1) Day of birth (31 April) is incorrect.
(2) Primary treatment has not been recorded.
(3) Site of first metastasis is other breast, visceral, or both.
(4) Age in completed years is inconsistent with the given dates of birth and of first treatment.
(5) Date of first metastasis has not been recorded, but site or sites of metastasis have been given.
(6) Date of death apparently precedes date of first treatment; the latter should probably be 1956 which would be consistent with age (in completed years) 36 at first treatment and survival (in completed years) of three years.
(7) Patient is recorded as alive *and* as having died from breast cancer.
(8) Code for fixation to the overlying skin is illegible.
(9) Ulceration implies international stage 3 breast cancer.
(10) International stage 2 disease denies ulceration.

Notice that mobile homolateral axillary nodes are consistent with international stage 2 disease and that regular menstruation is probable for a woman aged 36 years.

Reference to the hospital case notes would be necessary to resolve the above errors.

A computer program will often be written to check the integrity of clinical trial data. This check comes after a preliminary manual check; it follows the punching of the data and so can detect errors that have been introduced at that stage. Errors so detected are corrected by reference, in the first instance to the trial record sheets (in the case of punching errors, this will be sufficient) and thereafter to the doctor who completed the forms. It is the doctor who, knowing the case history, must resolve inconsistencies and retrieve missing data.

Comparability

(48) *Why is it necessary to check that the actual treatment groups are comparable on baseline characteristics even when the method of assignment is random?*

—randomisation does not guarantee balance in every instance; moderate discrepancy between randomised treatment groups with respect to baseline characteristics should be taken into account at analysis

—leak in randomisation suspected if groups not comparable?

COMMENT

Randomisation is expected to produce treatment groups that are comparable on important baseline characteristics but it will not do so in every instance, and so the investigator should check that a satisfactory balance has emerged. Not only the investigator but also the reader is reassured when there is no obvious initial discrepancy between the treatment groups. If there is a moderate imbalance then the author knows to take account of this in the analysis, and to check that there has not been a leak in the randomisation procedure.

Out of 28 prospective trials (*Lancet*: July to December 1977) that compared treatments between groups of patients, only 19 made a check on comparability; some imbalance was found in eight of the 19 studies.

References

1 Wilcox RG, Roland JM, Banks DC, Hampton JR, Mitchell JRA. Randomised trial comparing propranolol with atenolol in immediate treatment of suspected myocardial infarction. *Br Med J* 1980;**280**:885-8.
2 Henk JM, Kunkler PB, Smith CW. Radiotherapy and hyperbaric oxygen in head and neck cancer. *Lancet* 1977;ii:101-3.
3 Goebel KM, Goebel FD, Schubotz R, Hahn E, Neurath F. Levamisole-induced immunostimulation in spondyloarthropathies. *Lancet* 1977;ii:214-7.

The next step is analysis, and the next series on assessing methods answers questions about statistical methods commonly reported in medical journals.

ASSESSING METHODS—DESCRIPTIVE STATISTICS AND GRAPHS

In his 1981 presidential address to the Royal Statistical Society, Professor D R Cox said: "The setting out of conclusions in a way that is vivid, simple, accurate, and integrated with subject-matter considerations is a very important part of statistical analysis."

This series is about how to set out conclusions in medical papers and answers questions about when particular statistical methods are appropriate—and the hidden snags in using them. Types of problems that ought to be referred to a statistician are also discussed.

I shall review here descriptive statistics—mean, median, and mode, variance and interquartile range—explaining how a little detective work using these summary measures reveals a great deal about the distribution of observations even if a fully informative table or graph is not presented. It is usually helpful to use graphs to present data, and some reminders about how to do this are given—in particular, scattergrams are recommended.

(1) *From the table find the most likely (modal) survival time and estimate median survival for the 347 patients with breast cancer who were referred to the department of radiotherapy, Edinburgh, in 1956.*

—the most likely survival time is less than one year

—50% of patients survived for at least four years

—the difference (mean−median) is a crude measure of skewness

—measures of dispersion (variance, interquartile range) are needed to qualify central measures such as mean and median

COMMENT

Authors are advised to summarise important aspects of their data—location, dispersion, skewness—by reporting descriptive statistics such as mean, median, mode, variance, range, percentiles, but too often the summary is presented at the expense of informative tables or graphs. The reader is left to infer from the summary the shape of the underlying distribution. Some guidelines are given for doing this.

Measures of location (or centre) are mean, median, and mode. Mean and median coincide for symmetric distributions. The sum of the observations divided by the number of observations estimates the true mean, and the value above which 50% of the observations lie estimates the median of the distribution. When the estimated mean and median are dissimilar and sample size —which should always be reported—is moderate the reader can deduce that the underlying distribution is asymmetric or skewed. From the table notice that 174 (50%) of the 347 patients survived for at least four years after diagnosis of breast cancer. Mean survival exceeded seven years. The difference (mean−

Survival of 347 patients with breast cancer

Survival time (years)*	Frequency	Cumulative frequency
<1	62	62
1–2	45	107
2–3	38	145
3–4	28	173
4–5	25	198
5–6	10	208
6–7	14	222
7–8	11	233
8–9	9	242
9–10	8	250
10–11	8	258
11–12	8	266
12–13	9	275
13–14	5	280
14–15	2	282
15–16	3	285
16–17	4	289
17–18	7	296
18–19	1	297
19–20	3	300
At least 20	47	347

*The interval 1–2 years includes survival times of one year and up to, but not including, 2 years. All patients were followed up to the 20th anniversary of first treatment; 300 patients died before 31 December 1976.

median) is a crude measure of skewness. For breast cancer it is positive—three years—and allows the reader to infer that the distribution of survival time is positively skewed—mean survival is exaggerated by a small but important proportion of long-term survivors.

Survival for 347 patients with breast cancer: summary

q_1 = Lower quartile or 25th percentile

q_3 = Upper quartile or 75th percentile

The most likely survival time, however, is less than one year. More generally there may be several maxima, in which case the distribution is multimodal. A typical example of there being two modes (bimodality) is when anthropometric observations for men and women are combined. Shoe size—a crude measure of foot length—is shown below for a class of 49 undergraduates. There are two modes: shoe sizes 6 and 9 correspond to the mode for women and for men respectively.

Scattergram of shoe size for a class of 49 undergraduates

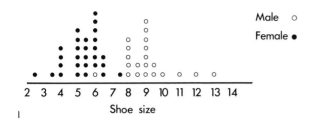

Measures of dispersion are variance, range, and interquartile range. They are needed to supplement measures of location.[1] An appropriate measure of dispersion should be reported alongside mean, median, or mode, just as sample size is needed for interpreting proportions or percentages. Variance is the average squared deviation from the mean and as such it—or standard deviation, which is the square root of the variance and is measured thus in the same units as the observations—is the best measure of dispersion when the mean is the best measure of location. When the underlying distribution is skewed it is important to qualify the median by reporting also the quartiles—above and below which 25% of the observations lie—or percentiles, such as the 10th and 90th. From the table we estimate that 25% of the 347 patients had died within 18 months after diagnosis of breast cancer and that for 75% of patients survival time was less than 11 years. The quartiles are shown in the figure.

How much of the information in the table is conveyed by the figure alone? The answer is a great deal if you follow the clues: the most likely survival time was less than one year, 25% of patients had died within 18 months of breast cancer having been diagnosed, and half within four years. Because mean survival is three years longer than the median survival time, the distribution of survival is positively skewed and so there are long-term survivors. Another pointer to positive skewness is the fact that the time interval between the upper quartile and the median—seven years—is considerably longer than the corresponding interval between the median and the lower quartile. Long-term survival is confirmed because 25% of patients were still alive 11 years after being treated for breast cancer.

(2) Mean survival was approximately five years for the 300 patients (see table above) who died before 31 December 1976. Why is it wrong to conclude that patients in Edinburgh with breast cancer have a mean survival time of five years?

—because the calculation ignored long-term survivors

—five years is therefore a serious underestimate of mean survival time from diagnosis

—in any case, median survival is a more reliable measure

COMMENT

Five years is an underestimate of mean survival time from diagnosis because the 47 patients excluded from the calculation were the long-term survivors—that is, they survived for at least 20 years. Since follow-up was discontinued at the 20th anniversary information on these patients is right-censored—that is, we know only that their survival times exceed 20 years. A better estimator is derived by crediting these patients with 20

years' survival and so obtaining
$$(300 \times 5 \text{ years} + 47 \times 20 \text{ years})/347 = 7 \text{ years}$$
as a more realistic measure, but an underestimate still because the actual survival times from diagnosis for these 47 patients must be *longer* than 20 years.

In these circumstances median survival is a more reliable measure of location than the mean because the survival distribution is skewed and there are incomplete lifetimes. It is also easier to find. Complete reporting of survival data entails plotting life-tables and is the subject of "Survival," page 82.

Another reason for being cautious is that if there is a time-trend in survival then patients referred in 1956 need not have the same survival pattern as patients referred more than two decades later. Patient care, or severity of disease, or treatment, or age at referral could have changed.

(3) Do figures A and B give the same information about tumour size?

—no, figure B is a misleading representation of the information given in figure A

—area represents frequency in a histogram

—neither figure mentions that tumour size was not recorded for 50 patients

COMMENT

Tumour size was measured clinically and rounded up to the nearest centimetre. Three patients had no measurable mass, and tumour size was not recorded for 50 out of 347 patients. Neither figure A nor figure B mentions these 50 missing observations. Figure A plots tumour size rounded up to the nearest centimetre, so that the 29 patients for whom recorded tumour size was 2 cm had tumours that measured more than 1 cm and up to 2 cm. Recorded tumour size is therefore on average $\frac{1}{2}$ cm more than actual size. Figure B purports to show the same data as figure A, but is misleading. The area of the bar over tumour size 10-15 cm represents a frequency of 40 patients—five times as many patients as really had a tumour that large. The bar over 15-20 cm is also in error by a factor of 5. Area, not height, represents

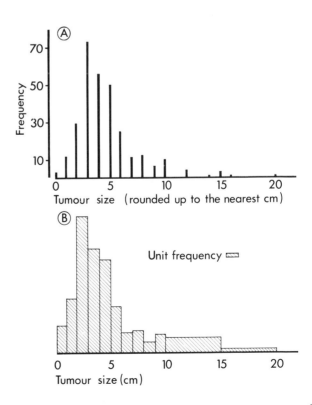

frequency in a histogram. In figure B, moreover, it is not possible to separate the three patients who had no measurable mass from the 12 patients whose tumour measured up to 1 cm.

(4) What is the minimum information that should be given with a graph?

—title, labelled axes, scale, key to symbols

—scattergrams are recommended for exploring and reporting data

—distinct points should represent distinct measurements; in particular, bilateral observations (ocular tension in right and left eye) should not be represented as unrelated

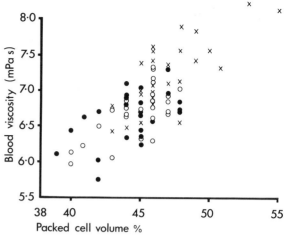

o Controls
• Patients with no stenosis or stenosis of one vessel only
× Patients with stenosis of two or three vessels

Blood viscosity and packed cell volume.
Conversion: SI to traditional units—Blood viscosity: 1 mPa s = 1 cP

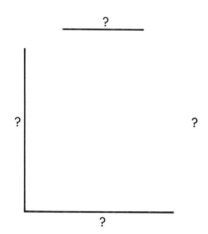

COMMENT

Graphs should have a title, axes should be labelled, and the scales given. Breaks in scale should be clearly marked and attention drawn to outlying or rogue observations. Healy[2] has written a good article on informal graphical methods for detecting rogue observations. Different symbols that appear in the graph should be defined in a key, or as a footnote to the graph. Lowe *et al*[3] studied the relation between the extent of coronary artery disease and blood viscosity in 75 men aged 30 to 55 years. Fifty men were studied before they underwent selective coronary arteriography for assessment of chest pain; the other 25 had been admitted for elective minor surgery and served as controls. In a single vivid scattergram Lowe *et al* showed comprehensively the association between packed cell volume and blood viscosity for the asymptomatic controls, for the patients with no stenosis or stenosis of one vessel only, and for patients with stenosis of two or three major coronary vessels. Scattergrams are an excellent device for exploring and reporting data, particularly for showing the association of one variable with another. Pocock *et al*[4] showed the negative association of standardised mortality ratio and water hardness in 234 towns in this way and also used maps to good effect to illustrate the findings of the British Regional Heart Study.

Editors often advise authors that graphs should be interpretable without referring to the text. This is a good maxim. Another important point is that repeated observations on the same patient should be identified on the graph as being related, and should certainly not be represented as though they were measurements on several different patients. If several similar plots are reported together comparisons can be made most easily if the scale and the symbols are consistent from one graph to the next. The choice of scale is important. Transformation of data is discussed next.

I thank G D O Lowe *et al* for permission to reproduce the scattergram under question 4.

References

[1] Gore SM, Jones IG, Rytter EC. Misuse of statistical methods: critical assessment of articles in *BMJ* from January to March 1976. *Br Med J* 1977;i:85-7.
[2] Healy MJR. The disciplining of medical data. *Br Med Bull* 1968;**24**:210-4.
[3] Lowe GDO, Drummond MM, Lorimer AR, *et al*. Relation between extent of coronary artery disease and blood viscosity. *Br Med J* 1980; **280**:673-4.
[4] Pocock SJ, Shaper AG, Cook DG, *et al*. British Regional Heart Study: geographic variations in cardiovascular mortality, and the role of water quality. *Br Med J* 1980;**280**:1243-9.

ASSESSING METHODS— TRANSFORMING THE DATA

Transformation is often needed to analyse medical data competently. There are four reasons for transforming data, but most often in practice a transformation selected for one purpose conveniently achieves the others as well. The reasons for transformation are as follows. (*a*) To arrange that the dispersion of coded observations is similar across all treatment or diagnostic groups[1]—so that changes in mean or median are not obscured by greater variability in some groups than in others. (*b*) To induce normality*—because many statistical tests such as Student's *t*-test require that the data are normally distributed. It is better to work with derived observations that have a Gaussian (normal) distribution than to use less powerful statistical methods on the untransformed data—for example, the logarithm of plasma cholesterol, being normally distributed,[2] could be compared between two groups of 20 patients each, say, using Student's *t*-test but not the plasma cholesterol concentration itself. (*c*) To produce simple relationships—the eye easily assimilates straight lines but is less good at detecting other patterns, such as quadratic, cubic, or exponential. By transforming one or both of a pair of variables an association can sometimes be presented as linear on the transformed data when it was more complicated on the original observations. (*d*) So that there is good agreement with biological or physiological principles—the plasma creatinine concentration indicates the level of renal function.[3] The kidney may be thought of as a sink or reservoir maintained at a constant level by drainage, and since the product of its input and output is constant the one is the reciprocal of the other, so that it makes sense to study reciprocal plasma creatinine as a monitor of renal function. The impressive work of Dr M S Knapp and his colleagues at the City Hospital, Nottingham in collaboration with Professor A F M Smith (Department of Mathematics, University of Nottingham), who have used reciprocal plasma creatinine to monitor the function of kidney transplants, shows that transformation is far from being a statistical nicety, it also has clinical relevance.[3] [4]

(5) *Which of the three plots shown in figures 1 and 2 gives the clearest indication of when rejection occurred in a patient who received a renal transplant?*

—reciprocal plasma creatinine concentrations corrected for body weight

COMMENT

Plotting plasma creatinine concentrations against time tells us little because as plasma creatinine concentrations decrease so, dramatically, does their variance. Plotted as in figure 1 the points therefore do not convey equal information, making the graph difficult to interpret. The need to transform the data was

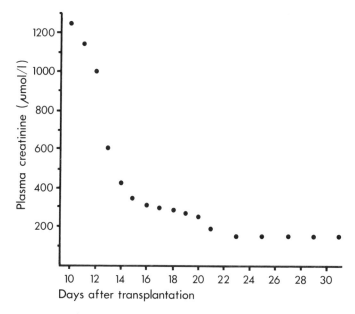

Rejection: day 24 approximately

FIG 1—Before transformation.
Conversion: SI to traditional units—Plasma creatinine: 1 μmol/l $\approx$ 88·4 mg/100 ml.

recognised because the distribution of plasma creatinine concentrations is highly skewed and by thinking about renal physiology. By plotting the reciprocal of plasma creatinine against time an abrupt change at approximately 24 days after transplantation for this patient becomes apparent. Because changes in plasma creatinine concentrations are caused by variations in the volume of distribution, which is commonly a result of fluid retention or diuresis, the Nottingham team first corrected plasma creatinine for body weight.[3]

The adjustment for weight is important (see figure 2) because the time of rejection now appears as the intersection of two straight lines having different slope. This simple representation, by no means obvious from figure 1, has been arrived at by carefully considering the statistical and physiological reasons for transforming the original observations. An interesting result of the Nottingham studies is that rejection is probably more common at night, having apparently a circadian rhythm, and is likely first to alter creatinine clearance at around 6 am.[4] The idea of making a correction for weight when concentrations are measured has been investigated also by Wald and his colleagues at Oxford.[5] They found that the maternal serum alphafetoprotein concentration is influenced by maternal weight and propose an appropriate adjustment. This type of transformation is likely to be generally important.

*Statistical distributions are discussed on page 94. This was not included in the original series but is published here for readers who are interested.

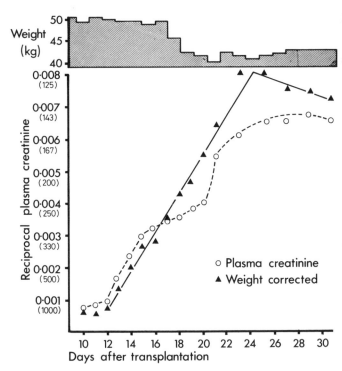

FIG 2—After transformation and correction for weight. The numbers in parentheses are plasma creatinine concentrations on the original scale of μmol/l—for example, 1 over 1000 μmol/l=reciprocal plasma creatinine, namely 0·001.

(6) *If asked to investigate an association between leucocyte count at initial assessment and subsequent survival time for patients with unresectable lung cancer, which transformations would you consider when plotting the data?*

—logarithmic transformation of survival time

—square-root transformation of leucocyte count

—when graphs are used to explore data the choice of the correct transformation is less important in practical terms than realising when some transformation is called for

COMMENT

When graphs are used to explore data the choice of the "correct" transformation is less important in practical terms than realising that "some" transformation ought to be tried and knowing broadly how to proceed. Mention of survival time should conjure up a picture of non-negative data skewed to the right, and the possibility that variance increases as mean survival time squared—which it does indeed if survival is exponential. Consideration should therefore be given to plotting the logarithm of survival time—the "correct" transformation when variance increases as mean squared, and a sensible approach when dealing with survival data generally, provided that survival times are not too close to zero. Likewise, mention of counts triggers the thought that as mean count increases so, as a rule, does the variance—making transformation appropriate. The "correct" transformation in this case would be the square root of the original counts, but taking logarithms instead—a more extreme transformation—will not usually do more harm than failing to transform the data at all.

As an aside I mention the logit transformation for proportions, which will be discussed in "Many variables," page 86. When plotting proportions—for example, of schizophrenic patients who develop tardive dyskinesia—against some risk factor, such as age or neuroleptic dose measured in equivalents of chlorpromazine, there may be need for transformation: because the

numbers at risk in different subgroups vary considerably or because the proportion of failures—that is, patients with tardive dyskinesia—ranges outside 0·30–0·7, wherein variance is relatively stable *provided* that the groups at risk are of similar size, or both. The reason for transformation is again to find a scale on which variance will depend neither on the estimated proportion nor on the number of patients in different groups at risk.

Reverting to the question of whether leucocyte count at initial assessment and survival time are associated for patients with unresectable lung cancer, all that remains is to plot for each patient the logarithm of survival time against the square root of leucocyte count and inspect the scattergram for evidence of association. Take care to distinguish between deaths and the survival times of patients who are still alive, using different symbols for exact (●) and censored (x) observations. The scattergram would be difficult to interpret if follow-up was incomplete on many patients so that censored observations were frequent, but this would be unlikely in a retrospective survey of patients with unresectable lung cancer. Life-tables have the advantage that they take proper account of censored survival times. An alternative plan, if sample size was moderate, would be to separate patients into three or more groups according to initial leucocyte count and to plot the life-table for each group of patients. The one difficulty here is deciding on the appropriate grouping. Any classification that is suggested by the data needs to be viewed cautiously and requires independent verification. A defendable solution is to group together the lower, middle, and upper-third of the distribution for leucocyte counts.

The suggestion[6] that the survival time of patients with unresectable lung cancer is related to initial leucocyte count was not supported by correspondents.[7][8] None of the authors published a scattergram for the information of readers, though Snell[7] had clearly constructed such a plot when exploring his data, and the observation by Huhti et al,[8] that high leucocyte counts were predominant only for patients who survived less than one month, could have derived from similar inspection. Publication of these figures would have needed little extra space and would have been more informative and less arbitrary than the original tabulation.[6] Authors should note that when transformed data are plotted or reported it is highly desirable to link the new observations to the original scale, providing, as it were, a translation for the reader into the language he is familiar with.

(7) *Tumour mass was measured clinically and recorded for 294 patients with breast cancer; the mean tumour size was 4·2 cm and standard deviation 2·7 cm. What do you infer from the above summary about the distribution of tumour size?*

—tumour size is not normally distributed

—there is a small proportion of very large tumours

COMMENT

If tumour size were normally distributed we should expect 95% of the observations to lie in the interval from approximately two standard deviations below the mean to roughly two standard deviations above the mean (the exact multiple is 1·96). This is the interval from $4·2-2\times2·7=-1·2$ cm to $4·2+2\times 2·7=9·6$ cm, but the implication that $2\frac{1}{2}\%$ of patients have tumour size *less* than "$-1·2$ cm" is clearly nonsense. The observations on tumour size are therefore not normally distributed (reductio ad absurdum); it is likely that the distribution is positively skewed, as indeed is the case (see table I). Some 60% of patients have tumour size less than 4·2 cm instead of the 50% we should expect from a Gaussian distribution.

How could we have derived a more sensible interval? The long upper tail to the distribution of tumour size points to a logarithmic transformation, although taking square roots gives a satisfactory enough answer (see table II)—better at least than

TABLE I—*Measured tumour size (rounded up to the nearest centimetre)*

Tumour size (cm)	Frequency (n = 294)
1	12
2	29
3	73
4	56
5	50
6	25
7	11
8	12
9	6
10	10
11	0
12	4
13	0
14	1
15	3
16	1
17	0
18	0
19	0
20	1

no transformation. The mean of $\log_e$ (tumour size) was 1·24 and standard deviation 0·66. The antilog of 1·24 is 3·5 cm, and the corresponding interval from two standard deviations below to two standard deviations above the mean—reported in the original units—is from antilog $(1·24 - 2 \times 0·66) = 0·9$ cm to antilog $(1·24 + 2 \times 0·66) = 12·9$ cm. Notice that this interval excludes the lower 4% and upper 2% of patients, agreeing

reasonably well with the expectation that about $2\frac{1}{2}\%$ would be excluded in each tail if $\log_e$ (tumour size) were normally distributed. Intervals calculated using logarithmic, square root, and no transformation are compared in table II, as are the observed numbers of patients whose tumour size exceeds the estimated 99th percentile—we should expect there to be three such patients. The interval derived using the logarithmic transformation is the best representation, in other words, $\log_e$ (tumour size) most closely of the three follows a normal distribution.

I am grateful to Dr M S Knapp and his colleagues at the Renal Unit, Nottingham and to Professor A F M Smith, Department of Mathematics, Nottingham University for permission to reproduce figures 1 and 2.

References

[1] Rogers K, Roberts GM, Williams GT. Gastric-juice enzymes—an aid in the diagnosis of gastric cancer? *Lancet* 1981;i:1124-5.

[2] Flynn FV, Piper KAJ, Garcia-Webb P, McPherson K, Healy MJR. The frequency distributions of commonly determined blood constituents in healthy blood donors. *Clin Chim Acta* 1974;**52**:163-71.

[3] Knapp MS, Blamey R, Cove-Smith R, Health M. Monitoring the function of renal transplants. *Lancet* 1977;ii:1183.

[4] Knapp MS, Cove-Smith JR, Dugdale R, MacKenzie N, Pownall R. Possible effect of time on renal allograft rejection. *Br Med J* 1979;i: 75-7.

[5] Wald N, Cuckle H, Boreham J, Terzian E, Redman C. The effect of maternal weight on maternal serum alpha-fetoprotein levels. *Br J Obstet Gynaecol* 1981;**88**:1094-6.

[6] Check IJ, DeMeester T, Vardiman J, Hunter RL. Differential counts and survival in lung cancer. *Lancet* 1978;ii:1317-8.

[7] Snell NJC. Leucocyte-counts and survival in unresectable lung cancer. *Lancet* 1979;i:383-4.

[8] Huhti E, Poukkula A, Saloheimo M. Leucocyte-counts and survival in lung cancer. *Lancet* 1979;i:1348.

TABLE II—*Tumour size: comparison of transformations*

Transformation	Interval representing the central 95% of tumour size distribution (cm)	Excluded		Estimated 99th percentile	
		Lower tail	Upper tail		Exceeded by (expectation: 3)
Logarithmic	0·9-12·9	4%	2%	16·0 cm	1 patient
Square root	0·5-10·2	2%	3%	11·5 cm	8 patients
None	−1·2- 9·6	0%	5%	10·5 cm	10 patients

ASSESSING METHODS—
ART OF SIGNIFICANCE TESTING

Statistical tests of significance make an important contribution in finding out whether differences between treatments are genuine. The first step is calculation—some theory and careful arithmetic tell us how probable is a result as extreme or more extreme than our observations, if there is actually no difference between the treatments. The art of significance testing comes with the second step—interpreting that probability (see page 18).[1-3] There is an EITHER/OR conclusion to a statistical argument, which is one very good reason why clinical decisions should not be made automatically on the basis of a single "statistically significant" finding—unless the significance level is very much more extreme than 0·05. Running major trials in parallel in different countries is recommended to expedite practical clinical decisions and to avoid ethical problems.

Interpreting significance tests calls for (a) good scientific judgment setting the results of this experiment in perspective: is the treatment a rational choice, are conflicting or corroborative reports of it already published, is the treatment effect accentuated in higher-risk patients; (b) awareness of what does not constitute good prima facie evidence: unexpected associations, benefit from treatment in an isolated subgroup only, improper repeated significance testing, and the danger that a publication bias favours positive findings; (c) complete reporting, including descriptive statistics (see page 64)[4] and estimation of the confidence interval (page 73). Estimating the interval ensures that non-significance is not mistaken for "no difference." Wide confidence limits are usually the hallmark of inadequate trials.

Two-tailed tests of significance predominate in medicine because the possibility of an experimental treatment being inferior cannot reasonably be excluded at the start of a clinical trial. The test region therefore comprises large positive or negative differences between treatments. Strong a priori grounds that favour one treatment indicate a one-tailed test of significance—looking for a treatment difference in a specified direction—but are also an ethical contraindication to a randomised clinical trial.

(8) *Interpret p <0·05 and p <0·01: given identical trial size, which gives stronger evidence against the (null) hypothesis that there is no difference between treatments?*

—if there is truly no difference between treatments an outcome as extreme or more extreme than that observed would occur fewer than: 5 times in 100 p < 0·05; 1 time in 100 p <0·01

—an outcome that would occur less often than 1 time in 100 when there is actually no difference between treatments is more extreme (that is, less compatible with the hypothesis of no treatment difference) than an outcome that arises perhaps as often as 5 times in 100.

COMMENT

Proof by contradiction is a major way of tackling logical and mathematical problems. Stating as his premise what he wants to disprove the logician argues correctly from that starting point and knows that if his arguments lead him to a contradiction then, since his method was correct, the premise must have been false.

In statistics we copy this approach but instead of reaching an absolute contradiction we observe an improbable outcome. Starting from a null hypothesis—that there is no difference between treatments, for example—we observe the result of a well-designed experiment, assess how likely the observed result is *from the standpoint of no treatment difference*, and if it is judged by a valid test procedure to be an improbable outcome then *either* we accept that there is really no difference between treatments and the improbable has happened—as it must occasionally do—*or* we argue that because the observed outcome is unusual (improbable) if there were no difference between treatments it is, on the contrary, plausible that there *is* a difference.

How large that difference is likely to be is reflected by the (confidence) interval from the smallest to the largest effect of treatment with which the trial data are consistent. That is to say if I took as my null hypothesis that the effect of treatment was any value in the quoted interval then my test procedure would not indicate that the result of the experiment was untoward.

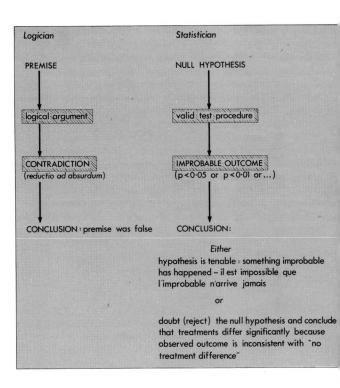

The *either/or* conclusion to a statistical argument explains why clinical decisions are not made on the basis of a single "statistically significant" finding, unless the significance level is very much more extreme than 0·05. Moreover, Zelen has warned that because authors and editors are reluctant to publish non-significant comparisons articles in medical journals may abound with false-positive claims—there are few really promising treatments and most comparisons are therefore made between

Clinical decisions are seldom made on the basis of a single "statistically significant" finding

equal contenders with only the 1 in 20 trials which fortuitously achieves p <0·05 being reported. Until editors insist on confidence intervals when publishing non-significant differences[2][5] rejoinders in the correspondence section are not the solution to Zelen's paradox. Non-significant findings from inadequate trials masquerade there as convincing counter-arguments because there is no obligation to report what are undoubtedly hopelessly

Editors should insist on confidence intervals when publishing non-significant differences

wide confidence intervals. Effective studies are undervalued and less informative than they might be because authors do not emphasise that narrow confidence limits mean precise estimation.

(9) What is evidence of a treatment effect or of association?

In addition to statistical significance on the credit side:

—treatment rationale

—dose-response relation

—effect of treatment evident in subgroups as well as in the trial as a whole

—epidemiological evidence

—more than one trial confidently pinpoints effect of treatment

—a single major trial and corroborative reports

On the debit side:
—an unexpected association needs to be checked with new data

—overall no significant treatment difference, but a significant effect in one subgroup

—eager and frequent perusal of accumulating data

Major trials should be run concurrently in different countries so that practical clinical decisions are delayed as little as possible

COMMENT

Statistical significance is necessary evidence but is not usually sufficient to change clinical practice unless one or more of the following conditions apply: (*a*) the treatment is a rational choice, fitting in with some theory about the disease process or because it has been shown to work for a related condition; or (*b*) a dose-response relation can be shown; or (*c*) the effect of treatment is evident in subgroups of patients as well as in the sample as a whole; or (*d*) epidemiological evidence can be adduced as in the report linking coffee and cancer of the pancreas[6]; or (*e*) more than one powerful clinical trial has been reported confidently pinpointing the treatment effect[7]; or (*f*) a single major trial has shown an overwhelming difference[8] and other reports—of related treatments or similar trial end points—are corroborative; or (*g*) combinations of these. Extra confirmatory evidence is needed because of the *either/or* conclusion to a statistical argument.

It is important also to recognise what is not good evidence. On the debit side therefore are the following. (*a*) An unexpected association, discovered only on careful scrutiny of the results and not one which the investigators were originally interested in. Such an association is that between coffee drinking and cancer of the pancreas. MacMahon *et al*[6] correctly emphasised the need for independent validation. (*b*) Clinical trials showing overall no significant difference between treatments but parading a significant effect in one subgroup of patients. Beware of multiple significance testing.[9] How many subgroups were examined? This information is important because fortuitously one group out of 20 will show a treatment effect (p <0·05), even when there is actually no treatment difference. Only an independent check will tell whether the treatment really is effective for this type of patient. (*c*) Eager and frequent perusal of accumulating data,[10] the authors reporting the moment that "statistical significance" is first achieved. The chance of finding p <0·05 at some time during a trial between equivalent treatments is close to 0·20,[7] whereas if up to 10 repeated significance tests are made using

A good general principle is to view sceptically the significance level p<0·05 if you suspect improper repeated significance testing

the criterion p <0·01 then the effective false-positive rate is still less than 0·05. A good general principle therefore is to view sceptically the significance level p <0·05 unless you can be sure that improper repeated significance testing is not responsible for it.

In relation to timolol in the treatment of patients after myocardial infarction Mitchell[11] asked: are consistent trends from many trials more convincing than a single trial with an extreme significance level such as p <0·001? The answer is twofold. Firstly, a proliferation of inadequate trials is bad science, and frequent repetition of major trials is unethical. The second answer lies in points *a* to *g* above of what is good evidence for saying that one treatment is superior to another. It is usually a matter of judgment whether further trials are needed. The tendency to publish only significant findings and to suppress inconclusive studies certainly distorts in the way that Zelen suggests—a disproportionate number of false-positives to be

> **Proliferation of inadequate trials is bad science; frequent repetition of major trials is unethical**

more expensive, but reluctant approval[11] of the results of the Norwegian timolol study and bewilderment over those of the clofibrate trial[12] convince me that vital questions merit this special attention. Perhaps Professor Mitchell's question may be rephrased to ask whether in future major trials should be replicated concurrently so that practical clinical decisions are delayed as little as possible.

sorted out by criteria *a* to *g*. There would be less need to exercise this type of judgment if only studies were published that are powerful enough to detect worthwhile and reasonable differences between treatments, irrespective of whether the outcome of such a trial is statistically significant, and if the practice of following the first positive result by a second trial for confirmation was replaced by a scheme that Dr A L Cochrane has advocated. Instead of one trial followed by another, if the two trials are devised concurrently and reported at about the same time by investigators from different countries then the probability that both will declare false-positives (p <0·05) is about one chance in 400, undistorted by publication or other bias. The method avoids ethical problems, gives a reassuring generality to the conclusions because they have been reached independently by different investigators, and is expedient because it does not delay acceptance of the findings by other doctors. In short, the proposal acknowledges that interpreting statistical significance is not always easy. Planning two trials instead of one is, of course,

References

[1] Peto R, Doll R. When is significant not significant? *Br Med J* 1977;ii:259.

[2] Rose G. Beta-blockers in the treatment of myocardial infarction. *Br Med J* 1980;**280**:1088.

[3] Altman DG. Statistics and ethics in medical research. Interpreting results *Br Med J* 1980;**281**:1612-4.

[4] Gore SM. Assessing methods—descriptive statistics and graphs. *Br Med J* 1981;**283**:486-8.

[5] Gore SM. Mexiletine after myocardial infarction. *Lancet* 1981;i:951.

[6] MacMahon B, Yen S, Trichopoulos D, Warren K, Nardi G. Coffee and cancer of the pancreas. *N Engl J Med* 1981;**304**:630-3.

[7] Peto R. Clinical trial methodology. *Biomedicine Special Issue* 1978;**28**:24-36.

[8] The Norwegian Multicenter Study Group. Timolol-induced reduction in mortality and reinfarction in patients surviving acute myocardial infarction. *N Engl J Med* 1981;**304**:801-7.

[9] Smith PG, Pike MC, Kinlen LJ, Jones A, Harris R. Contacts between young patients with Hodgkin's disease. *Lancet* 1977;i:59-62.

[10] McPherson K. Statistics: the problem of examining accumulating data more than once. *N Engl J Med* 1974;**290**:501-2.

[11] Mitchell JRA. Timolol after myocardial infarction: an answer or a new set of questions? *Br Med J* 1981;**282**:1565-70.

[12] Committee of Principal Investigators. WHO cooperative trial on primary prevention of ischaemic heart disease using clofibrate to lower serum cholesterol: mortality follow-up. *Lancet* 1980;ii:379-85.

ASSESSING METHODS— CONFIDENCE INTERVALS

Doctors understand so well the importance of checking whether an observed outcome is within the bounds of chance variation that the first two of three pithy definitions of god are as follows: the patient's definition is that the doctor is god, the doctor's definition of god is "$p < 0.05$," while the statistician. . . .

Careful reporting does not end at significance testing, especially when the author's summary is that the difference between treatments is not statistically significant ($p > 0.05$).[1] [2] What that amounts to is a statement that the trial results are consistent with there being no difference between treatments, and is not at all the same as saying that there is actually no difference. The distinction becomes clear if the authors report also the range from the smallest to the largest effect of treatment with which the trial data are consistent (see page 70)[3]—a 95% confidence interval, for example. This range includes zero when the difference between treatments is not statistically significant ($p > 0.05$) but accommodates also real positive and negative differences. If we assumed that the actual treatment effect is outside the quoted 95% limits and were to test the data from that viewpoint we would conclude that the outcome of the trial was improbable. Real differences of such magnitude are therefore confidently, though not definitely, excluded.[3] [4]

This is often a highly informative conclusion but is suppressed by mere testing of significance. Editors should encourage the reporting of confidence intervals for better communication of trial results and so banish for all time the mistake of identifying "not statistically significant" with "no difference."

(10) Is the treatment of patients with hypertension by trained industrial nurses a practicable alternative to treatment by the patient's family doctor? Four hundred employees with asymptomatic hypertension are randomised to care at the work site or a doctor's care, and the reduction in diastolic pressure is compared. The figure (A) gives an idea of the distribution of likely trial outcome if the two methods of treatment are equally successful. What conclusion do you reach if the actual trial outcome is (i) d_1; (ii) d_2; (iii) d_3?

(i) outcome d_1 is consistent with no difference between treatments: 95% confidence interval from -1.1 mm Hg to 2.5 mm Hg straddles zero

(ii) outcome d_2 is improbable ($p < 0.02$) if there is really no difference between treatments: 95% confidence interval from 0.4 mm Hg to 4.0 mm Hg indicates an advantage for treatment at the work site

(iii) outcome d_3 is highly improbable if there is really no difference between treatments: confirmation in the 95% confidence interval, which is from 2.0 mm Hg to 5.6 mm Hg

COMMENT

(i) Trial outcome d_1 is consistent with there being a small

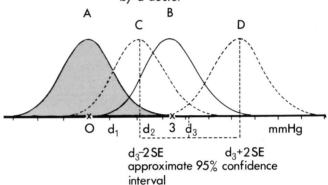

Treament of patients with hypertension at the work site or by a doctor

Horizontal axis is marked off from zero in units of 1 standard error (approx 0.9 mmHg)

A : Distribution of likely trial outcome when the 2 methods of treating hypertension are equally good

B : Distribution of likely trial outcome if care at the work site reduces diastolic pressure by a futher 3 mmHg

C : Distribution of likely trial outcome if care at the work site reduces diastolic pressure by a further 2.0 mmHg; outcome d_3 is not improbable $p > 0.05$

D : Distribution of likely trial outcome if care at the work site reduces diastolic pressure by a further 5.6 mmHg; outcome d_3 is consistent also with this distribution

difference or no difference at all between treatments. From this result we can be 95% confident that reduction in diastolic pressure under a doctor's care is neither better by more than 1.1 mm Hg nor worse by more than 2.5 mm Hg than monitoring by trained industrial nurses. Suppose that industry was prepared to offer treatment at the work site if the true reduction in diastolic pressure was 3 mm Hg more by this method than with a doctor's care. The clinical trial has provided useful information in so far as a differential of 3 mm Hg or more is confidently excluded. Had the industry's threshold been lower—2 mm Hg, say—no practical decision could have been reached, the outcome of the trial being consistent both with no difference and also with a difference of 2 mm Hg.

(ii) Outcome of d_2 is improbable ($p < 0.02$) if there is really no difference between the two methods of treating hypertension. The advantage of care at the work site is confidently estimated as anything from 0.4 mm Hg to 4.0 mm Hg. In particular, the trial outcome is not at odds with a real effect of 3 mm Hg diastolic pressure. If the confidence interval is uncomfortably wide for the decision maker then the trial should have been much larger. Four times as many patients are needed to reduce by half the width of the confidence interval.

(iii) The observed outcome d_3 is highly improbable, given that there is no real difference between care at the work site and a doctor's care. We are 95% confident that the advantage for treatment at the work site lies in a further change in diastolic pressure between 2·0 mm Hg and 5·6 mm Hg. This result would probably lead to providing trained industrial nurses to treat hypertension, but not necessarily so.

The example is based on an actual experiment in occupational health[5] and was devised so that there was at least a 90% chance of reporting statistical significance (p <0·05) if the real differential was as much as 3 mm Hg. If an industrial concern had been prepared to invest in treating patients with hypertension at the work site they would assuredly have required narrower confidence limits on the potential benefit. Precise estimation of the advantage of one scheme over another can be more persuasive than mere testing of significance. But in certain clinical trials pursuing randomisation beyond the point of having recognised that treatments differ significantly (p <0·01) would be considered unethical.

(11) What do you infer from the approximate 95% confidence intervals shown in the figure below about (i) trial size and (ii) treatments?

(i) the size of trial A is adequate to show convincingly the superiority of chemotherapy, that of trial B is needlessly large

(ii) multiple chemotherapy leads to a highly statistically significant increase in median survival time, which is also clinically relevant

COMMENT

Trial A roughly corresponds to the findings of Mallinson *et al*[6] who randomised 40 patients with inoperable cancer of the pancreas to multiple chemotherapy versus analgesic treatment (controls). Median survival was 44 weeks in the chemotherapy group, almost five times longer than for patients on the control arm. We can calculate confidence intervals for the ratio of the median survival in the chemotherapy group to the median survival in the control group by first calculating a confidence interval for the logarithm of the ratio—which is approximately normally distributed if the sample size is moderate and survival is exponential—and then transforming back. Two scales are shown in the figure. The lower is the exponential of the upper

scale: $1 = \exp(0)$ $3·3 = \exp(1·2)$ $11·0 = \exp(2·4)$ and so on. Notice that the confidence interval for $\log_e$ (ratio) is symmetric as usual, from 0·62 above to 0·62 below its midpoint 1·59, but taking exponentials gives an asymmetric confidence interval for the ratio of median survival times, the observed ratio 4·9 being closer to $2·6 = \exp(0·97)$ than it is to $9·2 = \exp(2·21)$. The confidence interval is approximate, given sample size.

Trial A and trial B (hypothetical) both indicate that median survival is significantly longer for patients who received multiple chemotherapy. From trial A we are 95% confident that median survival is at least 2·6 times longer in the chemotherapy group than for control patients who received only analgesics, and might be up to 9·2 times longer. Trial A does not estimate the ratio very precisely but it would have been wrong for the investigators to have continued to admit patients into a trial which had already shown an important effect of treatment—one sufficient to impress not only Dr Mallinson and his colleagues but other doctors as well. Historical data had not given reason to expect a dramatic effect of treatment and initially the authors had thought in terms of a larger trial. Trial B (hypothetical) reports a confidence interval that is only half the width of trial A's but required four times as many deaths to be observed. To have insisted on this greater precision would have been unethical. In the event, a smaller trial was adequate, the plans for a longer series being aborted.

(12) What do you infer from the approximate 95% confidence intervals shown in the figure below about (i) trial size and (ii) treatments?

(i) wide confidence intervals are associated with small trials: to reduce by half or one-third the width of a confidence interval needs four or nine times as many patients respectively;

the size of trial D is much too small; that of trial C is sufficient to give useful information

(ii) from trial C: there is 95% confidence that aspirin does not increase mortality by more than 0·7 deaths in every 100 patients

COMMENT

Trial C in this example—comparison of treatment with aspirin versus placebo in the prevention of secondary myocardial

Median survival (weeks)	Chemotherapy	Control	Ratio
Trial A	44	9	4·9
Trial B (hypothetical)	38	11	3·5

Confidence interval for ratio of median survival

Log_e(ratio)	-0·2 0	0·4	0·8	1·2	1·6	2·0	2·4	2·8
Ratio of median survival	0·8 1	1·5	2·2	3·3	5·0	7·4	11·0	16·0

( ) = confidence limits; x = point estimate

Chemotherapy versus analgesic treatment (controls) in patients with inoperable carcinoma of the pancreas: approximate 95% confidence intervals for the ratio of median survival time.

Percent dying	Placebo	Aspirin
Trial C	14·8	12·3
Trial D (hypothetical)	15·1	13·6

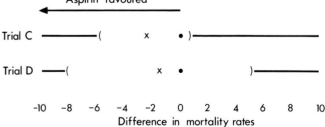

Confidence interval for difference in mortality rates

( ) = confidence limits; x = point estimate

Aspirin versus placebo in the prevention of secondary mortality after myocardial infarction: approximate 95% confidence intervals for difference in mortality rates at one year.

infarction—reproduces the results of Elwood and Sweetnam,[7] who randomised 1682 patients. The mortality at one year was not significantly lower in the group taking aspirin, zero being included in the approximate 95% confidence interval for the difference in mortality rates. But the interval conveys more information still. It permits the confident conclusion that an *increase* in mortality attributable to aspirin is no greater than an additional 0·7 deaths in every 100 patients, whereas the benefit could be as much as the prevention of 5·8 deaths. Trial D (hypothetical) can likewise be summarised by saying that treatments do not differ significantly ($p > 0.05$). The summary, however, obscures important differences between trials C and D. Firstly, by comparing the widths of the corresponding confidence intervals it is clear that the second trial entered only about one-quarter the number of patients randomised by Elwood and Sweetnam: the interval for trial D—from -8.4 to $+5.4$—having width 13·8 compared with 6·5 for trial C. The second point is that, although both intervals include 0, the confidence limits for trial D succeed only in excluding enormous differences between treatments that would not have been considered realistic anyway. For example, prevention of an excess of 8·4 deaths, more than half the expected mortality, would not have been thought within the capability of any drug a priori. Trial D has not increased our knowledge; trial C was an important and informative contribution, even though it did not show a statistically significant difference between the treatments.

Non-significant differences should not be dismissed just for having failed to reach conventional levels of significance. Confidence limits can advance our understanding; the width of the interval is a guide to how precisely or sensitively a parameter of interest, such as ratio of median survival times or difference in mortality rates, has been estimated. To show convincingly that for practical purposes two treatments are equivalent requires very precise estimation of the differential response, and hence very large numbers of patients.

References

[1] Rose G. Beta-blockers in immediate treatment of myocardial infarction. *Br Med J* 1980;**280**:1088.

[2] Gore SM. Mexiletine after myocardial infarction. *Lancet* 1981;i:95.

[3] Gore SM. Assessing methods—art of significance testing. *Br Med J* 1981; **283**:600-2.

[4] Armitage P. Statistical inference. *Statistical methods in medical research.* Oxford: Blackwell Scientific Publications, 1977.

[5] Logan AG, Milne BJ, Achber C, Campbell WP, Haynes RB. Worksite—treatment of hypertension by specially trained nurses: a controlled trial. *Lancet* 1979;ii:1175-8.

[6] Mallinson CN, Rake MO, Cocking JB, *et al.* Chemotherapy in pancreatic cancer: results of a controlled, prospective, randomised multicentre trial. *Br Med J* 1980;**281**:1589-91.

[7] Elwood PC, Sweetnam PM. Aspirin and secondary mortality after myocardial infarction. *Lancet* 1979;ii:1313-5.

ASSESSING METHODS—
RECOGNISING LINEARITY

Altman[1] has given a good account of the misuses of linear regression, noting that these are evident to the reader only if a scattergram of the data is published (see page 12). Examples of how to look at scattergrams are given here so that readers may develop a feel for correct applications and know how to recognise (*a*) when a regression function is non-linear, (*b*) when and why it is necessary to use weighted least squares, and (*c*) the danger of extrapolation beyond the data. Statisticians look first at a plot of the observations, judging from that the reasonableness of assuming a simple linear relation between the predicted and explanatory variable (with the attendant condition of constant variance about the regression line). I recommend this practice to doctors who want to explore their data carefully. The corollary is that for competent reporting of research findings authors should publish the relevant scatter plot—so that the method of analysis seems as obvious and convincing to the reader as it did to the investigators. Effective communication of results is a worthwhile goal after all.

Simple linear regression

(13) *Estimate from the linear regression function in the figure the expected reaction time for a surgeon whose heart rate is 90 beats per minute. Why is it unwise to use the figure for predicting mean reaction time when heart rate is 60 or 160 beats per minute?*

—the expected reaction time is 568 milliseconds

—the estimated linear regression function of reaction time on heart rate strictly applies only within the range of the observations; heart rates of 60 or 160 beats per minute are outside that range

COMMENT

Foster *et al*[2] reported significantly slower reaction time for surgeons whose heart rate while performing operations was lowered by oxprenolol. The outline for this example has some real basis, therefore, but the data in the figure are fictitious, as is the form—linear—of the regression function. The idea of a regression function is that it gives a formula for estimating the mean of the dependent variable (reaction time in my example) for given values of the explanatory variable (heart rate). This idea is illustrated in the figure, which, besides showing the scatter of the 50 pairs of observations, plots for intervals of heart rate— from the lowest to highest heart rate, grouping so that each interval has the same number of observations—the mean reaction time for surgeons whose heart rate fell in a particular interval against the corresponding mean heart rate. The symbols — in the figure lie approximately in a straight line with negative slope, giving the form of the regression function as reasonably linear.

It is important to remember that the regression function estimates the *mean* reaction time for a given heart rate. Different surgeons tested at this heart rate will record reaction times that centre on the estimated expectation but deviate individually in a

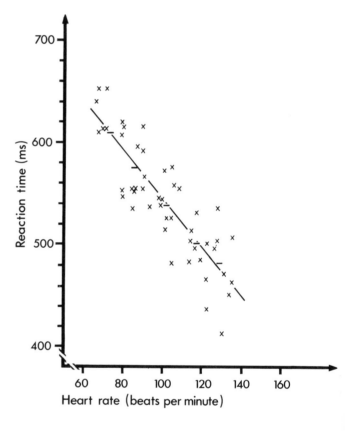

Simple linear regression function for mean reaction time given the heart rate (fictitious data). Interval means denoted by —. Residual variance $\hat{\sigma}^2$ is 830 sec².

The estimated regression line for mean reaction time is $783 - (2 \cdot 4 \times \text{heart rate})$. The estimator of mean reaction time given a heart rate of 90 beats per minute has a standard error of 5 milliseconds.

random fashion from it (as shown in the scatter plot). Testing the significance of and estimating confidence intervals for the parameters—slope and intercept for a linear regression function —are straightforward if we can reasonably assume that individual reaction times are normally distributed about their expectation.

From the figure we estimate that the expected reaction time is 568 milliseconds (standard error 5 ms) when heart rate is 90 beats per minute.

The evidence for linearity comes from the 50 pairs of observations reported in the figure. These observations are restricted to heart rates between 65 and 135 beats per minute, and statistical inferences should be similarly restricted for two reasons. Firstly, the idea that reaction time continues to slow by only 24 milliseconds for each further reduction of 10 beats in heart rate is ludicrous: in particular, reaction time would be infinite when there is no heart beat. Likewise, as heart rate increases beyond 150 beats per minute, quickening of reaction time would be cut short abruptly by some grave cardiovascular incident. Commonsense therefore warns against extrapolation beyond the range of the data. Secondly, there is an implicit statistical reason. The precision with which we estimate expected reaction time, given the heart rate, is less the further away the specified heart rate is from the centre of gravity of the observations. Imagine a hand as a fulcrum holding a rule which represents the estimated linear regression function. Errors in the estimation of intercept move the fulcrum up or down and errors of slope tip the ruler so that in combination they move the ends in a wider arc than points near the centre—a physical analogue of what happens in regression.

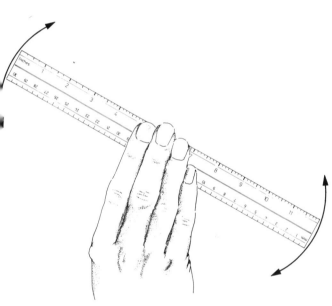

Physical analogue of linear regression.

Weighted least squares

(14) *The variance of reaction time is different in the figure according to heart rate. Describe how the variance changes, and say whether an observation $(80, x)$ gives as precise information about expected reaction time for a heart rate of 80 as the point $(120, x)$ conveys about the mean reaction time of surgeons whose heart rate is 120 beats per minute.*

—the variance of reaction time is greater when reactions are slow

—consequently an observation $(120, x)$ is a more precise estimator for mean reaction time given a heart rate of 120 beats per minute than $(80, x)$ is for the corresponding mean when the heart rate is 80

—weighted regression is called for because variance is not reasonably constant

COMMENT

Inspection of the scattergram in the figure (again fictitious data) shows fanning out of reaction times about the interval means. The dispersion is greatest when reaction time is slow and is least when mean reaction time is short. Such a picture is a denial of the assumption of constant variance and warns that simple regression methods are not appropriate. They, of course, are constrained to treat every paired observation as equally informative—reaction time having a random error component with the same variance irrespective of heart rate. Because reaction times are more widely dispersed when the heart rate is 80 beats per minute the analysis should give proportionally less weight to such observations. Statistical advice will usually be necessary to arrive at a correct analysis. What is important for readers and authors is being able to recognise when the method of weighted least squares is needed —and knowing the reason. I have explained the reason—

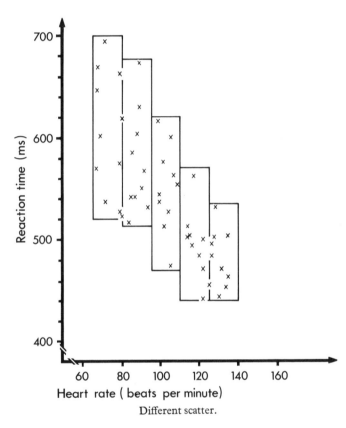

Different scatter.

heteroscedascity (from the Greek *hetros*, other or differently, and *skedannumi*, to scatter or disperse)—and suggested how inspection of scattergrams gives insight. Often, however, theoretical considerations hint at the correct analysis. Indeed, knowing that a surgeon's reaction time was measured by counting the number of responses in a two-minute interval and then dividing, I might have guessed that the distribution of counts was Poisson, making constant variance unlikely. A good example of statistical thinking being well illustrated is the work of Doll and Peto,[3] who related mortality (from smoking-related diseases) among doctors in different occupations to smoking ratio (a relative measure of cigarette consumption). The precision of the standardised mortality ratio (SMR) is known to depend on the number of deaths and was different for different specialties. Confidence intervals for the SMR were shown (see figure on next page), the longer confidence intervals that corresponded to groups with fewer deaths being given by broken lines to emphasise their unreliability and to focus attention on the shorter solid lines that denoted more reliable SMRs. This figure is an excellent representation for the reader of why the authors used weighted least squares to derive the regression line.

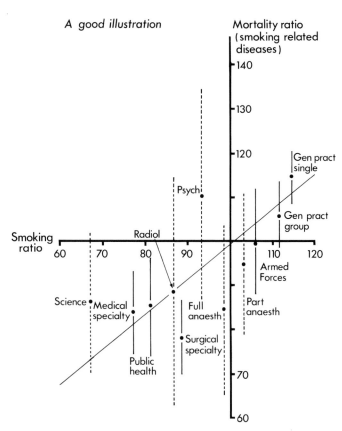

A good illustration

Standardised mortality ratio (SMR) (with 95% confidence interval) for mortality from main smoking-related diseases against smoking ratio for each of 11 specialties, together with regression line of SMR on smoking ratio. Longer confidence intervals corresponding to groups with fewer deaths are given by broken lines only to emphasise visually that they are unreliable and that attention should be directed chiefly to shorter solid lines, which describe more reliable SMRs.

I am grateful to Professor Sir Richard Doll and Mr Richard Peto for permission to reproduce their figure.

References

[1] Altman DG. Statistics and ethics in medical research. V Analysing data. *Br Med J* 1980;**281**:1473–5.
[2] Foster GE, Makin C, Evans DJ, Hardcastle JD. Does β-blockade affect surgical performance? A double blind trial of oxprenolol. *Br J Surg* 1980;**67**:609-12.
[3] Doll R, Peto R. Mortality among doctors in different occupations. *Br Med J* 1977;i:1433-6.

ASSESSING METHODS—
INITIAL IMPRESSIONS

Two examples of non-linear regression functions are given, only one of which can be transformed to become a straight line. Weighted least squares is again mentioned, and the idea of plotting interval means as a guide to the form of a regression function is emphasised in a second example.

Correlation coefficients make a useful contribution to preliminary data analysis only if supported by graphical methods. Authors are advised to report descriptively their initial impressions of complex data, giving the reader a useful background against which to see a final multivariate solution.

Non-linear relationships

(15) *Transformation*[1] *of one or both variables sometimes induces a straight-line relationship. Find the cube root of 0·125, of 1, of 8. What is the logarithm of 1, the square root of 4, the cube of 2, and the reciprocal of 2?*

—$0·125^{\frac{1}{3}}=0·5$; $1^{\frac{1}{3}}=1$; $8^{\frac{1}{3}}=2$

—$\log 1=0$; $\sqrt{4}=2$; $2^3=8$; $2^{-1}=\frac{1}{2}=0·5$

—**not all regression functions are linear**

COMMENT

The list of common transformations includes taking the logarithm, or the reciprocal, or the square root. The last two are particular instances of power transformations, $w=x^c$, the original variable x being raised to the power c. Taking $c=-1$ gives the reciprocal of x, and $c=\frac{1}{2}$ gives the square root. Transformation of one or both variables (explanatory or dependent, or both) sometimes induces a straight-line relationship. For example, figure 1 shows blood lead and first-flush water lead concentrations for 949 samples.[2] The non-linear relationship was shown using the technique that I described in question 13 (page 76).[3] Samples were allocated to nine groups of approximately 100, by water lead, and the group mean blood lead concentrations were plotted (see figure 2). The steep rise in blood lead concentration as water lead concentrations increased from 0·01 to 1 µmol/l levelled off at higher concentrations of water lead. Moore *et al* showed that the mean blood lead concentration tended to rise in proportion to the cube root of first-draw water lead concentrations so that transforming the explanatory variable in this case was sufficient to induce a straight line (see figure 3). The authors also noted from figure 1 that the variability and skewness in the distribution of blood lead concentrations were greater for high water lead concentrations, making weighted regression appropriate in addition to change of scale.

A second example of a non-linear relationship concerns the 1865 patients who survived for five years from a cohort of 3878 patients with breast cancer who were referred to the Western General Hospital, Edinburgh. The follow-up of these

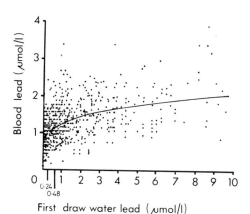

FIG 1—Scatter diagram for first-flush water.
Conversion: SI to traditional units—Blood lead: 1 µmol/l ≈ 0·0483 µg/100 ml.

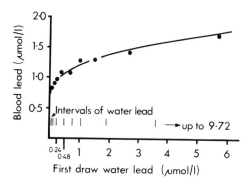

FIG 2—Mean blood lead concentrations for nine groups at intervals of first-flush water lead.

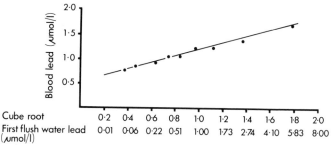

FIG 3—Interval means plotted against the cube root of first-flush water lead concentrations. Regression function linear.

patients and calculation of expected mortality has been described by Langlands *et al*.[4] Figure 4—the initial step in further

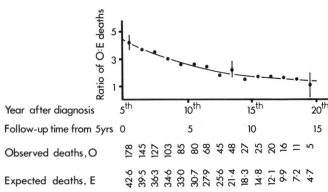

Observed deaths, O	178	145	127	103	85	80	68	45	48	27	25	20	16	11	5	
Expected deaths, E	42·6	39·5	36·3	34·6	33·0	30·7	27·9	25·6	21·4	18·3	14·8	12·1	9·9	7·2	4·7	

FIG 4—Five-year survivors (Western General Hospital breast cancer series). Ratio of observed to expected deaths and estimated non-linear regression function, $\beta_0 + \exp(\beta_1 - \beta_2 t)$. In three instances, 95% confidence interval for the ratio O:E is given to indicate reliability.

statistical modelling by Pocock and Gore of survival corrected for age—derives from that description. Note that the ratio of observed to expected deaths among five-year survivors falls from 4·2 in the first year of subsequent follow-up to 2·6 by the 10th year after diagnosis; and thereafter, because of the smaller numbers left, the ratio varied from year to year but remained greater than one. Approximate 95% confidence intervals for the ratio are shown in three instances to emphasise that the ratio is estimated less reliably in later follow-up. Weighted least squares is therefore appropriate. The ratio of observed to expected deaths diminishes, not linearly, but exponentially with length of follow-up and approaches an asymptote—a line which the curve continually approaches but never meets. The form of the regression function was therefore $\beta_0 + \exp(\beta_1 - \beta_2 t)$, the reasonableness of this form being shown in figure 4. It has the interpretation that if the asymptote β_0 is not significantly different from one, a proportion of breast cancer patients is cured. The actual results are not given here, my purpose being only to illustrate a case in which transformation could not induce linearity—taking logarithms does not help because β_0 gets in the way—and, incidentally, a further case which also needed to take account of ratios estimated with different reliabilities.

Authors must try to explain or interpret complicated regression functions if they hope to persuade the reader that the relationship is meaningful clinically as well as having a mathematical basis. Common sense and the need to convince others conspire together to put an effective ban on exuberant curve-fitting.[5] And rightly so.

Correlation coefficient

(16) The (Pearson) correlation coefficient is a measure of what sort of association?

—linear association

—correlation coefficients make a useful contribution to preliminary data analysis only if supported by graphical methods

COMMENTS

Altman[6] (see page 12) carefully distinguished between regression and correlation in presenting definitive results. I shall concentrate instead on preliminary or exploratory data analysis when the distinction is blurred in practice (without serious loss), the correlation coefficient being a convenient summary statistic provided that investigators (a) always inspect the corresponding scattergrams, (b) refrain from quoting significance levels when

describing this exploratory phase, and (c) include these initial impressions in a final report so that the reader can get a feel for the problem and understand why some variables but not others—either because they were too closely related or because they were uninteresting from the start—feature in a final statistical model. These remarks are illustrated with reference to the British Regional Heart Study.[5] (a) Two hundred and fifty-three urban areas were studied. Describing their *initial impression* of geographic variations in cardiovascular mortality, Pocock *et al*[5] listed the correlation coefficient with SMR (standardised mortality ratio for cardiovascular disease) for 24 factors, each of which had a marked association with cardiovascular mortality. But they also inspected scattergrams. There are two reasons for doing this. The first is to check whether the association is reasonably a straight line and if variance is well-behaved (constant)—departures from these ideals will modify later analyses. The scattergram of water hardness plotted against SMR was shown (figure). It suggested that the effect of water hardness was non-linear, being much greater in the range from very soft to medium-hard water than thereafter. This was verified later in a multifactorial solution that took account also of other variables, such as rainfall, temperature, and socioeconomic status.

The second reason for looking at scatter plots is to ensure that an important non-linear association—U-shaped, for example —which produces an insignificant correlation coefficient has not been missed, as it will be if the exploration goes no further than scanning correlation coefficients. No such associations were reported by Pocock *et al*, but there are plenty of examples

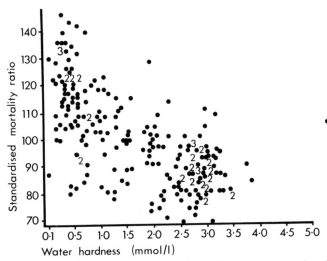

Water hardness plotted against standardised mortality ratio for all men and women aged 35 to 74 with cardiovascular disease for each town. (Water hardness: 1 mmol/l=calcium carbonate equivalent 100 mg/l.)

elsewhere—a U-shaped relation between weight and total mortality; a J-shaped relation of total mortality with plasma cholesterol concentration (for which an interesting explanation has been given[7]); and a non-linear association of alcohol consumption with mortality from all causes.[8] Therefore, do not rely only on correlation coefficients. (b) Looking at scattergrams and correlation coefficients one variable at a time against SMR gave only an outline description. This superficial view of the data may be considerably modified when several variables are taken into account together. Significance levels were not quoted for the 24 listed correlation coefficients because they would not reflect the relative importance of the different factors. Only a multivariate approach gives a solution to that conundrum. Emphasising this, Pocock *et al*[5] drew the reader's attention to the eight water variables among the 24 factors that showed a marked association with cardiovascular disease. Because the eight were highly dependent on each other, it was on the cards that they conveyed a single message—namely, some aspect of water quality is likely to be important. The message is made no more clear by quoting significance levels that are irrelevant when the real problem is multivariate. (c) The authors gained in the following respects by publishing their initial impressions. Firstly, the reader was acquainted with the complexity of variables—48 factors were considered as potential candidates in a multiple regression model for log SMR—and reasonably expected to see some of the 24 listed variables appearing in the final model. Because these 24 were grouped into categories—water, climatic, socioeconomic, geographical, blood group, air pollution—interest was focused on which categories stayed the course when there were many contenders instead of one, and also on how many representatives from each category were retained. Rainfall and mean temperature might offer different insights—both appeared in the final model—whereas because of their high interdependence the eight water factors might be adequately represented by one of their number, seen as a carrier for information on water quality generally. In a sense the preamble gave a forceful reminder that association is not causation. As the authors explained, total hardness was simply the water factor that they selected to show that the effect of water could not be explained away by other environmental factors such as rainfall. They could have shown this just as convincingly by using another of the eight—the concentration of water calcium, for example. Because the explanatory analysis was carefully described the reader could not fail to appreciate this point. A good general principle when reporting results is to take the reader through the steps the investigators made so that the reader is as comfortable with them as the authors are.

Correlation coefficients make a useful contribution to preliminary data analysis only if supported by graphical methods. Moreover, it is worth while for authors to report descriptively their initial impressions. I refer readers to an account by Altman[6] (page 12) for the sorts of error that occur when the significance of Pearson correlation coefficients is reported in definitive analysis. This test, as usually performed (under appropriate distributional assumptions), is made from the standpoint of no linear association[9] (see page 70)—a ridiculous standpoint when comparing, for example, two assays that purport to measure the same thing. Method comparison studies are discussed in some detail by Altman.[6]

To end with, an often repeated caution: statistical association is not, of itself, sufficient to impute causality to any observed relationship. How specific is the association—is water hardness related also to non-cardiovascular deaths?[5] Is the relationship consistent in time or with international studies, as the negative association of completed family size with mortality from ovarian cancer is?[10] Is there a possible mechanism? Is the apparent variable a proxy for some other—completed family size as a proxy for duration of breast-feeding, for example? How plausible is the alternative causality, such as proneness to ovarian cancer causing subfertility? St Leger et al,[11] who reported on factors associated with cardiac mortality referring particularly to the consumption of wine, warned against naively imputing cause. They were rewarded by a lively correspondence dealing with latitude,[12] milk,[12] sandwiches,[13] garlic,[14] and high-density lipoprotein cholesterol[15]—exemplary platelet activity.[16]

I am grateful to Dr Moore and colleagues for permission to use figures 1 and 2 and to Dr S J Pocock and co-workers for permission to reproduce the figure under question 16.

References

[1] Gore SM. Assessing methods—transforming the data. *Br Med J* 1981; **283**:548-50.
[2] Moore MR, Meredith PA, Campbell BC, Goldberg A, Pocock SJ. Contribution of lead in drinking water to blood-lead. *Lancet* 1977; ii:661-2.
[3] Gore SM. Assessing methods—recognising linearity *Br Med J* 1981;**283**:711-3.
[4] Langlands AO, Pocock SJ, Kerr GR, Gore SM. Long-term survival of patients with breast cancer: a study of the curability of the disease. *Br Med J* 1979;ii:1247-51.
[5] Pocock SJ, Shaper AG, Cook DG, et al. British Regional Heart Study: geographic variations in cardiovascular mortality, and the role of water quality. *Br Med J* 1980;**280**:1243-9.
[6] Altman DG. Statistics and ethics in medical research. Analysing data. *Br Med J* 1980;**281**:1473-5.
[7] Rose G, Shipley MJ. Plasma lipids and mortality: a source of error. *Lancet* 1980;i:523-6.
[8] Marmot MG, Rose G, Shipley MJ, Thomas B. Alcohol and mortality: a U-shaped curve. *Lancet* 1981;i:580-3.
[9] Gore SM. Assessing methods—art of significance testing. *Br Med J* 1981;**283**:600-2.
[10] Beral V, Fraser P, Chilvers C. Does pregnancy protect against ovarian cancer? *Lancet* 1978;i:1083-7.
[11] St Leger AS, Cochran AL, Moore F. Factors associated with cardiac mortality in developed countries with particular reference to the consumption of wine. *Lancet* 1979;i:1017-20.
[12] Segall JJ. . . . Milk. *Lancet* 1979;i:1294.
[13] Rao LGS. French wine and death certificates. *Lancet* 1979;i:1187.
[14] Slater NGP. . . . Or garlic. *Lancet* 1979;i:1294.
[15] Ricci G, Angelico F. Alcohol consumption and coronary heart-disease. *Lancet* 1979;i:1404.
[16] Manku MS, Oka M, Horrobin DF. Alcohol consumption and coronary heart-disease. *Lancet* 1979;i:1404.

ASSESSING METHODS—
SURVIVAL

The organisation and graphical representation of survival data are emphasised here. The comparison of lifetables using the logrank test[1] is recommended because it is more efficient than the comparison of survival rates at one point in time. Moreover, comparison of n-year survival rates can be misleading if investigators decide to make the comparison at a given time just because the observed difference is greatest then. Bad practice such as this does not escape notice if lifetables are necessarily reported.

Looking at lifetables readily suggests which factors are important for prognosis; plotting the rates of mortality year by year in addition to lifetables gives insight to the disease process and is the first step in assessing statistical models for describing survival. Diversity of times to peak hazard and the unimportance in later follow-up of prognostic factors that were relevant at the time of diagnosis may describe the pattern of mortality when there are long-term survivors, as in breast cancer.[2] Plotting the lifetable on a logarithmic scale is one method of assessing graphically whether survival is exponential. Other methods may be easier to interpret, however.

Organising survival data

(17) *Summarise the survival data at the time of analysis for patients A to D who were entered serially in a clinical trial comparing treatments for advanced cancer of the pancreas.*

—**patient A entered the trial on 14 January 1980 and was still alive at the date of analysis 30 June 1981, giving survival time of at least 533 days; the information that the patient died on 24 August 1981 is not available at the time of preparing the trial report**

—**patient B entered the trial on 31 January 1980 and died on 9 October 1980; exact survival time is 252 days**

—**patient C entered the trial on 27 February 1980 and was lost to follow-up on 1 April 1980, the latest date of contact with the patient; survival time for patient C is (right) censored at 34 days**

—**patient D was admitted to the trial on 16 August 1980 and was still alive at the date of analysis, though lost to follow-up later; being alive on 30 June 1981 means that the survival of this patient is (right) censored at 318 days, another way of saying that the patient's survival time is at least 318 days**

—**at the time of analysis survival is (right) censored for patients A, D, and C because patients A and D are still alive and patient C was lost to follow-up; survival time is exact for patient B, who has died**

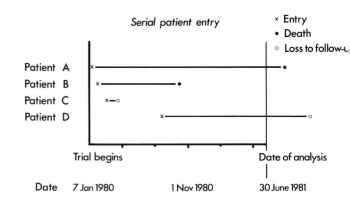

COMMENT

The following discussion is about time to death, but the event that is most important could as well be tumour regression, development of metastasis, rehabilitation after a stroke, reinfarction, discharge from hospital, or regaining birth weight for a preterm infant. Several of these events are less easily defined than death, so that in practice the study may be more difficult but in principle the same type of information is being recorded —namely, the time from entering the study to the occurrence of the particular event.

In most clinical trials patients enter serially—in the order in which they are referred. The first step in organising survival data, after fixing the date for analysis, is to update the follow-up on all patients so that each case history is summarised by only one of the following three descriptions. Description (1): patient died before analysis on —— (give the date, and cause of death if inferences about competing risks are to be made). Description (2): patient is "known" to be alive at the time of analysis (presumption is not good enough, because of the possibility of bias). Description (3): latest date before analysis on which the patient was known to be alive is —— (give date and reason for information being incomplete, such as the patient is abroad or no reply has been received to letters requesting follow-up information or the case notes have been mislaid, etc). The next step is to check that the sequence of dates is correct for a given patient and also that trial numbers and entry dates correspond. Any inversion— such as patient 12 was entered on 2 May 1981 while patient 13 was entered earlier on 16 April 1981—suggests an error in transcribing dates or in the trial procedures. Having checked the orderliness of the data, the third step is to convert dates into survival time in days. Survival time is exact for patients who have died and is right-censored for patients who satisfy descriptions (2) and (3), these patients having survived for a time of *at least so many days*. The information is now in a form that makes it straightforward to estimate the lifetable for different treatment groups as they were randomised and to compare the duration of survival, using, for example, the logrank test. An excellent guide to the comparison of lifetables has been published by Peto *et al*.[1]

Censored survival times are dealt with easily when computing lifetables (experimental survival curves) for different treatment groups. We assume, however, that the reasons for censoring are independent of treatment. If this is not so the comparison of lifetables could be biased. In particular, ensure that the follow-up of patients who have been withdrawn from treatment—because of toxicity, for example—is as intense as for patients who continue on treatment. The former group may be disadvantaged also in terms of survival, so that if toxic reactions occur more often in one treatment group failure to follow-up such patients shows that group in a relatively better light than is

Design and analysis of randomised clinical trials requiring prolonged observation of each patient:
Introduction and design   Br J Cancer 1976; 34:585-612
Analysis and example   Br J Cancer 1977; 35: 1 - 39
R Peto et al

warranted. Notice also that the detection of a local recurrence, say, or metastasis tends to be earlier when the interval between follow-up visits is short, so that routine appointments should be arranged similarly for all treatment groups. The reasons for censoring are important even when estimating a single lifetable as the following example shows. In the Western General Hospital breast cancer series,[2] patients were dismissed from follow-up at the 20th anniversary of first treatment if there was no recurrent disease. Patients who continued to be followed up after the 20th anniversary had an unfavourable prognosis therefore, and the duration of their survival would be a poor reflection of the outcome for all 20-year survivors. Langlands et al[2] avoided potential bias by censoring survival at the 20th anniversary for *all* patients in the Western General Hospital breast cancer series.

Certified cause of death is often unreliable in cancer series because deaths from other causes are underreported,[3] a proportion of them being described as deaths from cancer. When analysing overall survival all deaths are accounted for irrespective of the cause. One justification for this type of analysis is that what is important to the patient is life. To assess curability, however, it is useful to have some measure[2]—such as the excess death rate or the ratio of observed to expected deaths—which allows for the normal mortality in the general population. In one sense, therefore, death from cancer and death from other causes are competing risks. Analyses of duration of survival corrected for age and the study of curability and of competing risks are problems that should be referred to a statistician.

Lifetables and annual rate of mortality

(18) *Figure 1 shows the lifetable for breast cancer patients referred to the Western General Hospital, Edinburgh in 1956. Estimate the probability that a patient referred for treatment of breast cancer survives for 10 years or more from date of diagnosis.*

—for any time t, the lifetable gives the estimated probability of surviving for at least time t

—always plot survival data as a lifetable (another name for the lifetable is Kaplan-Meier experimental survival curve)

—plot also the annual proportion dying, which is related to what statisticians call the hazard function

—28% of patients with breast cancer survive for 10 years or more from date of diagnosis

COMMENT

A simple identity gives the principle on which calculation of lifetables is based. The identity is that the probability of surviving for (t+1) days from diagnosis equals *the probability of surviving for t days, multiplied by the probability of surviving the next day.* The last term, the probability of surviving day (t+1), is got by counting (a) how many patients are at risk (t+1) days after diagnosis—only patients whose recorded survival time is (t+1) days or more are in the group at risk; (b) how many patients died on day (t+1); and then computing (c) the probability of surviving that day as *one minus the proportion who died*—the proportion who died being the number of deaths on day (t+1) divided by the number of patients in the group at risk. Notice that the lifetable is a step function that estimates

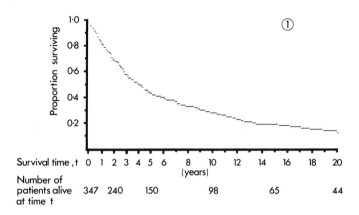

Lifetable for 347 patients with breast cancer referred to the Western General Hospital, Edinburgh.

the true survival curve in an unbiased way and that steps occur only at times of death. Readers are referred for a worked example and further explanation to the expository paper by Peto *et al.*[1] This gives sound advice about the design[4] and analysis[1] of randomised clinical trials that require prolonged observation of each patient.

By plotting the lifetable authors report survival data more completely than by summarising 5-year and 10-year survival rates. The lifetable gives for any time *t* in the range of the observations the estimated probability of surviving for at least time *t*. In addition, comparison of lifetables gives a preliminary impression of which factors are important for prognosis. Figure 2 shows that international stage separates patients with

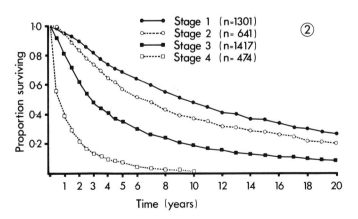

breast cancer into four groups with progressively poorer survival —69% and 57% of patients with stage 1 and 2 breast cancer survive for five years or more compared with 35% of patients with stage 3 and 7% of patients with stage 4.

Lifetables are not the only graphical representation of survival data and, because they show cumulative information, questions about how the rate of mortality changes year by year cannot be answered directly—although the answers are implicit in figure 2. I have in mind questions such as this: is the relative disadvantage of stage 3 breast cancer as great 15 years after diagnosis as it was at five years? The solution is to plot for each year of follow-up or other interval covering a sufficient number of deaths the estimated proportion of those alive at the beginning of a year who die within the year. To ensure proper handling of censored survival times, derive these proportions from the lifetable—for example, 41% of stage 3 patients survived for four years and 35% for five years, making the estimated proportion who died in the fifth year of follow-up equal to 6/41=0·15, or 15% (see figure 3). Obvious from figure 3 but concealed in figure 2 is

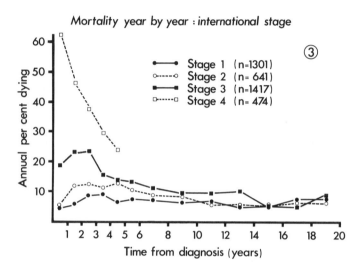

that the rate of mortality decreases for stage 4 patients: more than 60% die within one year of diagnosis. For patients with international stage 1, 2, or 3 breast cancer a different pattern emerges. Hazard increases during the first one to four years after diagnosis and then slowly declines. Peak hazard is not only greater but also occurs earlier in stage 3 and stage 2 disease. By the 10th year after diagnosis the annual percentage dying is similar for survivors from all three stages—remembering that a standard error qualifies the estimators. In particular, survivors from stage 3 breast cancer seem to experience the same rate of mortality at 15 years after diagnosis as do survivors from stages 1 and 2.

Reference points for choosing a description of survival are exponential survival (constant annual proportion dying), the Weibull family (risk of dying is monotone—it increases (or decreases) steadily from time of diagnosis), and the proportional hazards model[5] (irrespective of the elapsed time since diagnosis the ratio of the risks of dying in given prognostic groups remains constant, in particular the time when the force of mortality is greatest is the same for all prognostic groups). The problem of fitting a parametric distribution to survival needs to be referred to a statistician, but an initial assessment can be made from figure 3. The annual proportion dying is neither constant nor monotone and so the exponential model and the Weibull are not in the running. Diversity of times to peak hazard and the relative unimportance in later follow-up of description of the tumour (international stage) that was relevant initially are a denial of the proportional hazards model. These features suggest that a log-logistic distribution might fit the data. Careful statistical analysis is called for to substantiate these impressions.

When analysing long-term follow-up of patients investigators should plot mortality year by year in addition to the cumulative proportion of patients who survive. They should be on the look out for prognostic factors which, although relevant at diagnosis, are less important when it comes to describing later follow-up. Variable time to peak hazard indicates accelerated failure in some groups compared to others.

Look out for prognostic factors which, although relevant at diagnosis, have less importance when it comes to describing later follow-up

(19) *If the graph of log p_t (where p_t is the estimated probability of surviving for t years or more) plotted against time is a straight line then the survival distribution is exponential. What do you infer from the figure below about the survival of patients with breast cancer?*

—**survival is not exponential**

—**rate of dying for breast cancer patients as a whole is rapid during the first four to five years after diagnosis; thereafter the annual proportion dying is less, but moderately constant**

—**the hazard pattern for important subgroups of patients (according to international stage, for example) is different from the pattern for the series as a whole**

COMMENT

The figure shows the lifetable from figure 1 in question 18 plotted on a logarithmic scale. I have mentioned already that the exponential distribution is one reference standard for survival data—a particularly simple one, the time-specific risk of dying

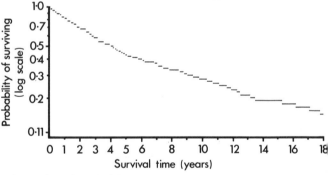

Distribution of survival in 347 patients with breast cancer referred to the Western General Hospital, Edinburgh.

or hazard being constant irrespective of the elapsed time since diagnosis. This means that the rate of mortality neither intensifies nor mitigates at any time during follow-up. Fairly simple statistical theory tells us that if survival is exponential, then the graph of log p_t against time looks like a straight line. For any other survival distribution a similar theoretical exercise indicates the appropriate transformation of p_t, which induces a straight-line relationship and so gives a visual test of goodness of fit. The exponential example is most familiar, however. The slope or gradient is identified with the rate of mortality, which is most intense when the gradient is steepest.

The difficulty of translating from gradient to hazard is avoided in figure 3 in question 18 by plotting annual mortality directly. The logarithmic plot is the more commonly reported, however, and so I include an example of it though it is not the method that I favour.

From the figure we see that the rate of dying is rapid and probably constant during the first four to five years after diagnosis—by placing a ruler along the line of the early part of the slope observe the more gentle gradient in the later part of the graph. This lies above the ruler and approximates to a different straight line. Our conclusions are (a) that survival is not exponential, and (b) that the rate of dying does not increase for the series as a whole. Recall, however, the initially increasing mortality associated with international stage 1, 2, and 3 breast cancer (see figure 3 under question 18). It is not unusual for the pattern of mortality in subgroups to be different from the overall impression. Investigation of prognostic factors should include looking at graphs of mortality plotted year by year.

Inefficient or misleading comparison

20) Comment on the comparison of survival at the fixed times shown in the figure below.

—comparison of three-year survival rates misses the emergent difference between treatments A and B

—comparison of two-year survival rates favours treatment A, whereas by seven years after diagnosis the advantage is with patients randomised to treatment B; the logrank test would identify neither treatment as superior

COMMENT

Comparison of n-year survival rates is inefficient because it ignores the structure of the lifetable and is open to the criticism that if the time of analysis had been chosen differently the results might be slanted differently. Peto *et al*[1] list comparison of survival rates at one point in time as the first of 13 bad methods of analysis. Avoid comparison of n-year survival rates.

The inefficiency of this method is illustrated in the figure on the left. By comparing three-year survival rates a difference between treatments that becomes apparent in time is missed. Comparison of lifetables over the entire follow-up period by the logrank test makes efficient use of the data and is likely to identify the superiority of treatment B.

In the second example, on the right of the figure, the treatment that is singled out as advantageous is different at two years and seven years. Treatment B is associated with higher initial mortality. In this case the logrank test is likely to report no significant difference between treatments. Only by plotting lifetables will the investigator discover the cross-over of the survival curves, an unusual contingency in practice—one that the logrank test does not deal with happily, nor does any other simple test statistic.

A third example, not illustrated, is when an initial treatment advantage (in the first year, for instance) is not sustained thereafter. This means that the rates of mortality in the two treatment groups are likely to cross-over, being first higher in one treatment group and then in the other before approaching a common level. Significant difference in disease-free interval but not in overall survival is the guise in which this problem commonly presents.[6] Statistical advice should be sought.

Comparison of n-year survival rates is at best inefficient, at worst misleading. Unless lifetables are plotted the two extremes cannot be identified separately. Organising survival data to compute lifetables and calculation of the logrank statistic are so much the same exercise that there is little justification for presenting an inferior analysis—and lifetables should of course be reported always.

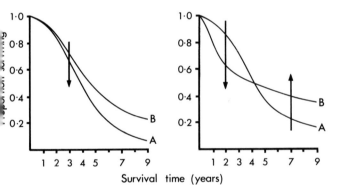

Survival time (years)

Undesirable comparisons of survival rates.

References

[1] Peto R, Pike MC, Armitage P, *et al*. Design and analysis of randomized clinical trials requiring prolonged observation of each patient. II Analysis and examples. *Br J Cancer* 1977;**35**:1–39.

[2] Langlands AO, Pocock SJ, Kerr GR, Gore SM. Long-term survival of patients with breast cancer: a study of the curability of the disease. *Br Med J* 1979;ii:1247–51.

[3] Cutler SJ, Axtell LM, Schottenfeld D. Adjustment of long-term survival rates for deaths due to intercurrent disease. *J Chron Dis* 1969;**22**:485–91.

[4] Peto R, Pike MC, Armitage P, *et al*. Design and analysis of randomized clinical trials requiring prolonged observation of each patient. I Introduction and design. *Br J Cancer* 1976;**34**:585–612.

[5] Palmer MK, Hann IM, Jones PM, Evans DIK. A score at diagnosis for predicting length of remission in childhood acute lymphoblastic leukaemia. *Br J Cancer* 1980;**42**:841–9.

[6] Henk JM, Kunkler PB, Smith CW. Radiotherapy and hyperbaric oxygen in head and neck cancer. Final report of first controlled clinical trial. *Lancet* 1977;i:101–3.

ASSESSING METHODS—
MANY VARIABLES

Seeing a way through many variables is an exciting challenge. By making the best use of latent information a whole range of problems can be solved—screening patients for referral to a hypothyroid clinic[1]; predicting the outcome for a patient with severe head injury so that limited resources for intensive care are used constructively[2]; identifying before operation patients at high risk of developing postoperative deep vein thrombosis[3] (for whom prophylactic heparin is justified); explaining variation in cardiovascular mortality[4] and making diagnoses[5] [6]; ensuring that clinical trial results are not distorted by chance imbalance between randomised treatment groups[7]; or setting up a prognostic staging system that accords with survival.[8] Doctors who have identified such a problem in their own specialty are advised to consult a statistician about the details of analysis, which may be fairly complicated. The simple underlying principle is to combine some or all of the many explanatory variables as a descriptive, predictive, diagnostic, or prognostic index for the appropriate outcome or dependent variable.

A second class of problems—for example, understanding how a disease presents—leads to the analysis of multi-way contingency tables, and statistical consultation is again advised.

(21) *Identify a common structure for the five problems shown in table I and suggest why the methods of analysis differ in detail but not in principle.*

—in each of the five problems there is a set of predictor or explanatory variables, some or all of which will be combined to explain, predict, or describe the dependent or outcome variable

—methods of analysis differ in detail because of (i) restrictions on scale for the outcome variable (probabilities are constrained to be in the interval [0,1], the risk of dying is non-negative); (ii) choice between an additive or multiplicative model (subject matter and the data usually determine which is more appropriate); (iii) requiring the random error terms in the statistical model to have constant variance to avoid the need for weighted regression

—the principle behind multivariate methods should be illustrated in a table or graph that shows how successful the predictions are in relation to the observed outcome

—ideally the success of any statistical model should be tested on new data

COMMENT

Inferences from any method of analysis are reliable only when the data have been collected in a disciplined way, the series of study patients being in some defendable sense repre-

sentative. Data from clinical trials generally satisfy this require‐ ment because the entrance criteria define the study population; a series of consecutive patients is acceptable provided that there is no important seasonal variation or other time trend either in the presentation of the disease or its outcome that would preclude making general inferences. Authors should recognise and comment upon the limitations of their sample. They must try to assess how these limitations might promote or eliminate particular variables in an explanatory model.

Many variables seem at first to be a matrix of insufferable complexity, but simple summaries and illustrations can be used to good effect[9] (see page 79) to give an initial impression of predictor variables and to group together those that are highly interdependent. This is the foundation on which any multi‐ variate statistical model is built. The next step is deciding the form of the regression function and whether the outcome variable needs to be transformed to induce a particular structure of error. Statistical advice is usually necessary. In practice, predictors are most often combined linearly, as in the five examples that follow: when the outcome variable is transformed to control variance linearity often comes as a by-product. The examples are in order of increasing technical difficulty as regards estimating the coefficients in the prediction equation—a statistical problem. A reporting problem is that the transformed scales on which it is convenient and reasonable to perform statistical analyses are less familiar in examples (3) to (5) than in examples (1) and (2). Authors should communicate their findings by mentioning the methodology briefly but concentrate on the clinical inter‐ pretation and applicability of the results in language that is familiar to readers. A good example is the description by Clayton et al[3] of a predictive index for postoperative deep vein thrombosis. The common thread in the five examples is the combining of several explanatory variables to describe or predict an outcome. Keep that idea firmly in mind and the barrier of transforming the problem for analytic reasons becomes trivial. Also good reporting should emphasise the clinical interpretation of results, and how they should be used— to help decision making or for test reduction.[6] It is important for doctors to recognise when methods, as described here, might be applied in their specialty and to seek statistical collaboration on what are often exciting and challenging problems—statistically as well as clinically.

(1) Mean heart rate during operation[10] depends on the surgeon's age and seniority, resting heart rate, the type and length of the operation, scrub-up time, medication (such as beta-blockade), and so on. The problem is to combine some or all of these explanatory variables in a prediction equation for mean heart rate during the operation to give a better under‐ standing of their relative importance. The outcomes for individual surgeons will, of course, deviate randomly from the predicted means, and this accounts for the error terms that bedevil statistics. Suppose that mean heart rates from 80 to 140 beats per minute have been observed. Possibly the residual random variation increases with the increase in predicted mean heart rate, but in the first instance constant variance could be assumed. Common sense suggests that a reasonable form for the prediction equation is a baseline mean heart rate β_0, which is modified up or down by adding weighted terms (the coefficient

TABLE I—*Problems with a common structure*

	Outcome variable				
	(1) Surgeon's mean heart rate during operation	(2) (Logarithm of) standardised mortality ratio for cardiovascular disease	(3) Postoperative deep vein thrombosis	(4) Tardive dyskinesia: absent, mild, moderate, severe	(5) Risk of dying after myocardial infarction
Explanatory or predictor variables, some or all of which are selected:	Age Seniority Specialty Smoking habit Length of operation Scrub-up time Resting heart rate Beta-blockade	Total water hardness Rainfall Maximum temperature % manual workers Car ownership	Age % overweight for height Preoperative stay Cigarette smoking Varicose veins Malignant disease Fibrinogen Factor VIII as % of normal Euglobulin lysin time Serum FR antigen	Age group Inpatient/outpatient status Dose of antipsychotic drugs (chlorpromazine equivalents) Duration of treatment Anticholinergic medication Parkinsonism Sex	Timolol/placebo Sex Age group Previous infarction Angina Treated hypertension Diuretic treatment before admission Beta-blocker treatment before admission Heart failure Lowest systolic blood pressure <100 mm Hg Arrhythmias in acute stage Site of infarct Smoking habit

$\beta_1, \beta_2, \ldots \beta_8$ are the weights) to account for age, seniority, length of operation, and so on. If one or more of the weights is not significantly different from zero then the corresponding explanatory variable might be eliminated from the prediction equation without serious loss of predictive value. Selecting a small number of explanatory variables is a non-trivial statistical problem. (The availability of statistical packages on computers does not lessen the need for statistical thinking. Blunderbuss approaches to statistical modelling are wasteful.) A multiple regression model for predicted mean heart rate during operation combining explanatory variables linearly has the form

$$y_{x_1, x_2, \ldots x_8} = \beta_0 + \beta_1 x_1 + \beta_2 x_2 + \ldots + \beta_8 x_8$$

where y denotes predicted mean heart rate.

(2) Pocock et al[4] noted that water hardness and other factors have a proportional effect on cardiovascular mortality. That is to say, if towns A and B are similar in all respects except water hardness (0·2 mmol/l in town A and 1·3 mmol/l in town B, say) then the SMR (standardised mortality ratio for cardiovascular diseases) for town B is expected to be 8% less than in town A, so that if town A's SMR is 100, town B has SMR=92, whereas if town A has SMR of 150, town B's SMR will be 138. This is what we mean by a constant *proportional* effect of water hardness on SMR. A multiplicative (proportional) model for SMR is equivalent to an additive model for log SMR and so Pocock et al used the logarithm of SMR as the dependent variable in a multiple regression model. The dependent and explanatory variables are different from those described in the multiple regression model above but transforming the outcome variable has induced the same structure, and the method of analysis is the same thereafter. Figure 1 shows actual SMR against predicted SMR, prediction being based on the set of five explanatory variables in table I. The authors noted that some towns, especially in Scotland, had a higher cardiovascular mortality than the model predicted, and this geographical clustering in mortality is being investigated. Departures from a predicted model, as in this case, often suggest new lines of research. The performance of a regression model should always be reported—on a familiar scale—so that readers as well as authors appreciate the relevance of the modelling.

(3) A simple prognostic index for predicting before operation which patients will develop postoperative deep vein thrombosis was established by Clayton et al[3] using clinical and coagulation data obtained before operation on 124 patients, of whom 20 had thrombosis. The structure of this problem is similar to the previous examples but the emphasis—identification of high-risk patients—is different and the technical detail more difficult. In the original 124 cases a binary outcome was observed (presence or absence of postoperative deep vein thrombosis) and we want to predict, for future patients, a probability. Directly predicting the probability of postoperative deep vein thrombosis for a given type of patient is troublesome for two reasons: firstly, because variance depends on the estimated probability, and secondly, a predicted probability outside the

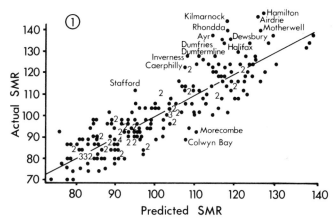

Actual SMR for cardiovascular diseases plotted against SMR predicted from five-variable model for 234 towns.

interval [0,1] would be nonsensical. Both these difficulties are avoided by translating the problem into predicting the log odds which has an unrestricted range—the conversion between the log odds (logit) and probability scales is shown in figure 2. (The log odds scale is one of several on which proportions can be analysed.) Clayton et al called the log odds scale the *predictive index*. The five out of 10 variables that they identified as having the best predictive power gave the following index

$$I = -11 \cdot 3 + 0 \cdot 009 x_1 + 0 \cdot 22 x_2 + 0 \cdot 085 x_3 + 0 \cdot 043 x_4 + 2 \cdot 19 x_5$$

where x_1 = euglobulin lysis time (minutes), x_2 = concentration of fibrin-related antigen (mg/l), x_3 = age (years), x_4 = percentage overweight for height, and x_5 = presence or absence of varicose veins (scored as 1 or 0 respectively).

High positive values of the predictive index are associated with a high risk of developing postoperative deep vein thrombosis. In a prospective study of 62 new cases,[11] using a cut-off point of −2 correctly identified nine out of 10 patients and incorrectly identified seven out of 52 patients as being at risk of developing postoperative deep vein thrombosis (see figure 3). This discrimination was as good as that obtained on the original data. Validating prediction models on the original data, which they were designed to reproduce, gives an overoptimistic view of their performance. Only by testing models on new data is their worth firmly established.

(4) Kidger et al[12] described a scoring system for orofacial and neck movements in patients with psychiatric illness. By grading the total score to give close agreement with doctors' rating of tardive dyskinesia each patient was allocated to one of four ordered categories: tardive dyskinesia—absent, mild, moderate, or severe. The next question is whether factors such as age, duration of treatment, dose of antipsychotic drugs (measured in chlorpromazine equivalents), Parkinsonism,

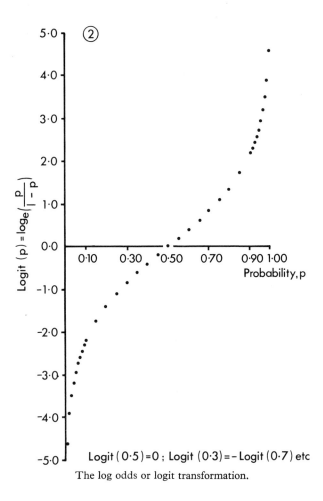

Logit (0·5) = 0 ; Logit (0·3) = – Logit (0·7) etc

The log odds or logit transformation.

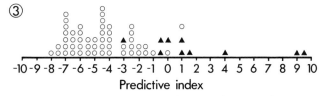

Distribution of preoperative predictive indices for the 62 patients studied

○ Patients who did not develop deep vein thrombosis
▲ Patients who did develop deep vein thrombosis

anticholinergic medication, inpatient/outpatient status etc, in some combination partially explain severity of tardive dyskinesia. An extension of the logistic model in example (3)—appropriate when the outcome variable is an ordered category—might be the method of choice. Intuitively a graded or ordered outcome is more informative than collapsing scores to give a crude classification: tardive dyskinesia—absent or present.

(5) Patients were randomised after myocardial infarction to timolol or matched placebo.[7] By chance—assuming no randomisation leak—the placebo group includes a higher proportion of patients aged 65 years or older, patients with arrhythmias in the acute stage, patients with a clinical history of treated hypertension, or patients who had taken diuretics. Of course, these variables are interrelated, older patients being more likely to have arrhythmias in the acute stage and to have been on diuretic treatment before admission, but it will be important to check that a definite effect of treatment persists after allowing retrospectively for moderate imbalance between the groups as randomised. Attention focuses on the time-specific risk of dying or hazard, a convenient measure of the changing force of mortality in time. If we assume a proportional hazards model —a reference point that is not always valid[13] (see page 82)—then

we claim that there is a basic form of hazard which is pr portionately increased or decreased according to the set explanatory variables which describes a particular patient.

The constant of proportionality is most often taken to be th *exponential* of a linear combination of the explanatory variables—exponentiation being to ensure that the final estimates a non-negative. Whether the patient was randomised to timolo would be included as one of the explanatory variables and if th treatment effect were still significant after adjustment for ri factors as described above, then the investigators would b reassured that the advantage was probably genuine and not a artefact because of moderate imbalance between the randomise groups.[7] It is certainly not the case, as Mitchell suggests,[14] tha an imbalance in risk factors, significant at the 1% leve necessarily translates into a survival difference, significant als at the 1% level. What the implications for survival are may b sorted out by an analysis of the type described above. Perhap Professor Mitchell's whimsical account was intended as a rebuk against the failure to report fully a sophisticated analysis?

Regression models for survival can be adapted to give prognostic classification of patients as in childhood acu lymphoblastic leukaemia[15]—using proportional hazards—c breast cancer.[8]

Fairly complex statistical methods have been discussed i relation to the problems in this commentary. Complexity is n always necessary. Comparing statistical techniques in th context of diagnosing hypothyroidism, Gardner and Barke concluded that a simple method—counting the total number symptoms present—was as effective in determining a rule fe

> Complexity is not always necessary
>
> Common sense should not be divorced from statistical thinking

referral as more complicated methods. Thomson *et al*[16] modifie a predictive index for which patients should be asked to giv consent for mastectomy because they wanted to avoid mammo graphy in younger women.

Common sense should not be divorced from statistica thinking.

(22) *Calcium as a measure of water quality was not included i the five-variable regression model for log SMR reported b Pocock et al.[4] Does this mean that water calcium is irrelevar as an explanatory variable for cardiovascular mortality?*

—**no**

—**excluded variables are superfluous, not irrelevant**

COMMENT

The results of Pocock *et al*[4] do not imply that the variable excluded from the prediction are useless indicators of cardio vascular mortality. The implication is rather that, after takin account of the information already in the prediction equatio the remaining variables are redundant in the sense of nc adding anything further to the explanation. A different regressio model—in which water calcium replaced total water hardnes as a measure of water quality—could have been propose

> Regression models give an explanation not *the* explanation: selection of predictor variables requires judgment as well as technical expertise

without serious loss. Regression models give an explanation not the explanation, because selection of predictor variables requires judgment as well as technical skill.

(23) There is recent evidence from another clinical trial that treatment A is more successful in male patients. How would you expect the statistician to allow for this in a regression model that takes account of several risk factors?

—by including an interaction term

COMMENT

The effect of treatment A would be measured by two indicator variables, one pointing to male patients, the other to female patients. If the corresponding estimated coefficients were significantly different the effect of treatment A probably differs between the sexes. Interaction terms are not convincing unless there is a sensible interpretation of them, or prior justification for their inclusion. Doctors should advise the statistician if they have good reason to suspect that a treatment will be more effective in one group of patients than another.

(24) Tumour size, fixation/ulceration, clinical disease of the homolateral axillary nodes, and presence/absence of other signs associated with poor prognosis) were recorded for 3695 of the 3922 patients in the Western General Hospital breast cancer series. Table II—a cross-classification of patients by these clinical features—shows part of the data. How many patients with no other signs were referred with tumour size 5 cm or more, no fixation to the overlying skin, and no nodal disease?

—74

—analysis of multi-way contingency tables leads to general inferences about how disease presents

COMMENT

Analysing the completed four-way contingency table (table II) answers questions such as: Is tumour size larger when there are other signs present? Does increased tumour size mean more disease in the homolateral axillary nodes? Does the apparent association of tumour size and fixation resolve if we take into account the state of the axillary nodes? Is there an important second-order interaction of fixation/ulceration, nodal disease, and presence/absence of other signs, for example?

These questions are not answered satisfactorily by considering only two factors at a time. A statistician would usually be consulted about the analysis of multi-way contingency tables. The usefulness of this approach is that it leads to general inferences about how a disease such as breast cancer presents.

I am grateful to Dr S J Pocock and colleagues for permission to reproduce figure 1 and to Dr A J Crandon and others for figure 3 under question 21.

References

[1] Gardner MJ, Barker DJP. Diagnosis of hypothyroidism: a comparison of statistical techniques. *Br Med J* 1975;ii:260–2.

[2] Teasdale G, Parker L, Murray G, Knill-Jones R, Jennett B. Predicting the outcome of individual patients in the first week after severe head injury. *Acta Neurochir* 1979;suppl 28:161–4.

[3] Clayton JK, Anderson JA, McNicol GP. Preoperative prediction of post-operative deep vein thrombosis. *Br Med J* 1976;ii:910–2.

[4] Pocock SJ, Shaper AG, Cook DG, et al., British Regional Heart Study: geographic variations in cardiovascular mortality, and the role of water quality. *Br Med J* 1980;280:1243–9.

[5] Bouckaert A. Computer diagnosis of goitres. III Optimal subsymptomatologies. *J Chron Dis* 1971;24:321–7.

[6] Card WI, Emerson PA. Test reduction. I Introduction and review of published work. *Br Med J* 1980;281:543–5.

[7] The Norwegian Multicenter Study Group. Timolol-induced reduction in mortality and reinfarction in patients surviving acute myocardial infarction. *N Engl J Med* 1981;304:801–7.

[8] Myers MH, Axtell LM, Zelen M. The use of prognostic factors in predicting survival for breast cancer patients. *J Chron Dis* 1966;19:923–33.

[9] Gore SM. Assessing methods—a feel for other things. *Br Med J* 1981;283;775–7.

[10] Foster GE, Evans DF, Hardcastle JD. Heart-rates of surgeons during operations and other clinical activities and their modification by oxprenolol. *Lancet* 1978;i:1323–5.

[11] Crandon AJ, Peel KR, Anderson JA, Thompson V, McNicol GP. Post-operative deep vein thrombosis: identifying high-risk patients. *Br Med J* 1980;281:343–4.

[12] Kidger T, Barnes TRE, Trauer T, Taylor PJ. Sub-syndromes of tardive dyskinesia. *Psychol Med* 1980;10:513–20.

[13] Gore SM. Assessing methods—survival. *Br Med J* 1981;283:840–3.

[14] Mitchell JRA. Timolol after myocardial infarction: an answer or a new set of questions? *Br Med J* 1981;282:1565–70.

[15] Palmer MK, Hann IM, Jones PM, Evans DIK. A score at diagnosis for predicting length of remission in childhood acute lymphoblastic leukaemia. *Br J Cancer* 1980;42:841–9.

[16] Thomson HJ, Miller SS, Gore SM, Bayliss A. Consent for mastectomy. *Br Med J* 1980;281:1097–8.

TABLE II—*Cross tabulation by clinical features*

	Other signs absent: fixation/ulceration			Other signs present: fixation/ulceration		
	1	2	3	1	2	3
Nodes 1						
Size 1	249	160	4	7	12	1
2	206	531	9	12	103	10
3	74	242	13	16	131	50
Nodes 2						
Size 1	83	69	0			
2	118	305	10			
3	45	174	11			
Nodes 3						
Size 1						
2						
3						

Factor	Coding	
Tumour size	Size ≤2 cm	1
	3–4 cm	2
	≥5 cm	3
Fixation/ulceration	No fixation, no ulceration	1
	Fixation, no ulceration	2
	Ulceration	3
Homolateral axillary nodes	Not affected	1
	Mobile	2
	Matted	3

ASSESSING METHODS—
CRITICAL COMMENT

To end this series I present mistaken examples from medical journals. Readers are asked to identify oversights in the design of these studies, misuse of statistical methods, or careless interpretation of results. I have not tried to find a comprehensive set of examples—good scientific method, frank reporting, and careful refereeing should make that task difficult—but there are enough cases to remind us to be critical in appraising research papers, even if they have passed an editorial filter. This will ensure that we learn and propagate the best methods. Errors in analysis do not necessarily invalidate conclusions,[1] and careless interpretation can be reviewed by correspondents. Faults in the design of a clinical study are not easily remedied after the event. This is why statisticians primarily emphasise good scientific method.

Having no wish to pillory the papers which inspired these examples, I am grateful to Dr Tony Smith, deputy editor of the *BMJ*, who provided parodies of the original versions. The examples contain the original fallacy, but the medical context has been changed.

(25) *Comment on the analysis (implicit in the figure below) of increased temperature gradient after withdrawal after one year of the β-blocker olalol in 12 out of 29 consecutive patients.*

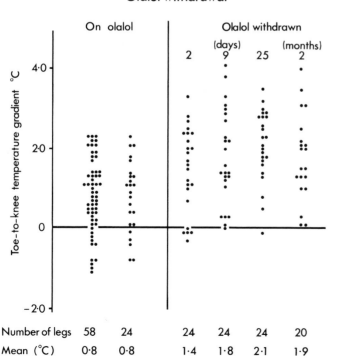

Olalol withdrawal

| Number of legs | 58 | 24 | 24 | 24 | 24 | 20 |
| Mean (°C) | 0·8 | 0·8 | 1·4 | 1·8 | 2·1 | 1·9 |

—**17 patients refused to approve withdrawal**

—**distinct points in the figure do not represent distinct patients**

—**from the figure it is impossible to deduce for individual patients the change in temperature gradient after withdrawal of olalol**

—**there is no randomised control group**

—**temperature gradient was measured knowing that treatment had been withdrawn**

—**patients who refused were not followed up**

—**two volunteers were lost to follow-up, with no explanation, at two months**

COMMENT

The refusal of 17 patients to take part in the study identifies them as different from the patients who agreed to forego medication. The similarity of the initial mean temperature gradient for volunteers and non-participants does not negate this essential difference. In the figure notice that it would have been better to show the scatter of initial temperature gradient for patients who refused than to present data on the combined group, of which volunteers are a subset.

The distinct points in the figure do not represent distinct patients. Temperature gradients in the right and left leg of the same patient tend to be more similar than such observations on randomly chosen patients. Failure to analyse correctly dependent observations is an error of commission[1]: the figure misleads the reader into thinking that the study is more informative than it is. Repeated measurements—as in right and left leg—lead to a better estimation of temperature gradient for a patient, but that is all. They do not increase the number of individuals in the sample.

The change in temperature gradient for individual patients cannot be deduced from the figure because the several measurements made in one patient are not shown as being related. The mean change is, of course, easily computed as the change in means, but the standard error required for Student's paired *t*-test— valid only if the change in temperature gradient is normally distributed—cannot be estimated from the data given. When statistical method and the figure are unrelated, as here, authors should draw attention to this and explain why the data are so represented.

Olalol was withdrawn in all patients who agreed to take part in the study and the authors reported that toe-to-knee temperature gradient increased as a result. The increase cannot logically be attributed to the withdrawal of medication because at the same time as olalol was withdrawn other changes had occurred coincidentally. One particular change was that the patients entered a clinical study, which might in itself account for the observed difference in temperature gradient, making treatment irrelevant. Had patients been randomised to olalol or matched placebo during the study and had there been a significant increase in temperature gradient for the placebo group relative to patients randomised to continued medication, the authors' conclusion could have been confidently made, but not in the absence of a randomised control group.

The patients understood the nature of the study because they gave informed consent, and the assessor was therefore unlikely to have remained in the dark. Knowing that treatment had been withdrawn may have biased the measurement of the temperature gradient. The accusation of bias cannot be refuted. This shows up the experimental design as imprudent.

Not only was there no randomised control group, but the temperature gradient was not measured in the patients who continued to take olalol, having refused its withdrawal. Patients who refuse should be followed up in the same way as patients who give consent. If temperature gradient increased also in patients who persisted with β-blockade, a suspicion that some unexpected time trend might account for the results would be reinforced. A cautionary tale about before-and-after comparisons has been reported by Christie.[2] Avoid this type of comparison because the inference is uncertain.

Finally, no explanation was given by the authors for the loss to follow-up at two months of two out of the 12 volunteers. Did these two revert to β-blockade and, if so, why?

(26) *Does the advice about drinking fewer cups of tea follow directly from the analysis below?*

—no

—a prospective study in which patients are randomised to receive or not receive encouragement to drink fewer cups of tea could give direct evidence

COMMENT

The relative risk of subarachnoid haemorrhage for women who reduce their tea drinking from more than four cups a day to

---

Tea drinking and deaths from subarachnoid haemorrhage

Analysis
The overall matched pair risk ratio (R·R) between current tea-drinkers and non-tea-drinkers was 1·9 (95% confidence interval 1·5 to 2·4)
For drinkers of fewer than 2 cups a day the relative risk was 1·2
At a level of 2-4 cups a day the relative risk was 2·3
And for drinkers of 5+ cups a day the relative risk was 4·0

Conclusion
These results suggest that the heaviest drinkers could halve their risk of death from subarachnoid haemorrhage by reducing their tea consumption to an intermediate level ; and that benefit of a similar order would be experienced by drinkers of 2-4 cups a day who cut down to less than 2 cups daily

---

between two and four cups a day may be quite different from the relative risk for women who never drank more than four cups of tea a day. An increased relative risk in association with drinking more cups of tea is not sufficient to determine cause. For instance, women who are at high risk of developing subarachnoid haemorrhage may drink more tea because of this. Reducing their intake would not alter the underlying risk factor. Since the authors do not give the relative risk, even for women who have chosen to drink fewer cups of tea than previously, their conclusion, however plausible, remains mere speculation. The theory that subarachnoid haemorrhage will be less frequent in patients who have been instructed to drink fewer cups of tea can be tested formally by randomising patients to receive or not receive advice about reducing tea consumption.

(27) *Is the evidence in the box below sufficient to recommend the self-treatment of warts with vinegar?*

Self-treatment of warts with vinegar was described in the medical news column of a women's magazine. Readers who tried the method were encouraged to write and say if it was successful. Thirty letters were received in four months, 25 from readers who said that the method had worked spectacularly. No reader wrote to say that the method was tried but had failed

---

—no

—readers who tried the method and failed to find relief were not motivated to write about it

COMMENT

The method's success rate could be estimated only if every reader who tried treating warts with vinegar had written to the magazine. Even then the population of patients could not be defined and the rate of spontaneous remission is unknown. This means that the success rate for self-treatment of warts with vinegar cannot be shown to be better than spontaneous remission.

The "experiment" is even more anecdotal because the magazine will not receive letters from every reader who tried self-treatment with vinegar. I suspect that readers who tried the method and failed to find relief were not motivated to write about it. This being the case, not even the treatment's rate of success could be estimated from the reports that the medical columnist has received.

(28) *Does the correspondence in the box refute the earlier report that survival is significantly longer for women than for men with rectal cancer?*

—no

—although the difference in survival is not statistically significant in the second series, median survival times are similar to those in the original report

—statistical significance depends on the number of patients studied as well as on how different the survival of men and women with rectal cancer really is

—a real improvement of $2\frac{1}{2}$ months in median survival may not be enough to justify antiandrogen treatment for men

---

First report : Median survival for 127 women with rectal cancer was significantly longer (p<0·01) than for 116 male patients, half of whom died within $4\frac{1}{2}$ months of diagnosis

Correspondence : The records of 72 unselected patients with rectal cancer were reviewed. There were 39 men and 33 women. Mean age at diagnosis and treatment for metastatic disease were similar; median survival (6 months for women, $4\frac{1}{2}$ months for men) was not significantly different between the sexes

---

COMMENT

The authors of the first report on 243 patients were surprised to find that survival was significantly longer for women than for men with rectal cancer and suggested that the observation needed to be checked in other series. If substantiated, a clinical trial of antiandrogen treatment for men patients would follow.

A second series of 72 patients with rectal cancer was reported. The correspondent noted that median survival was not significantly different between the sexes. Median survival times were, however, similar to those in the original report—a point that was not made in the letter to the editor. Statistical significance depends on the number of patients studied as well as on how different the survival characteristics of men and women with rectal cancer truly are. If the survival pattern were indeed the same in the two series and survival could be assumed to be exponential, then there is only a 40% chance that by investigating 72 patients the survival difference between men and women would be statistically significant. The second report is therefore not at odds with the outcome in the original series, the second investigation having low power.

Whether an expected improvement of $2\frac{1}{2}$ months in median survival is of sufficient clinical importance to warrant a randomised controlled trial of antiandrogen treatment for men is a decision for doctors to take. Statistical significance is of no account.

(29) *Comment on the data presented in the table and on the comparison of means using Student's paired t-test.*

—**variance is not constant; the three measures of outcome need to be transformed before using classic tests**

—**for the first two outcomes, response to exercise and the number of anginal attacks in two weeks, the standard deviation increases in proportion to the mean, indicating that a logarithmic transformation is appropriate**

—**the variance of trinitrin dose increases in proportion to the mean dose and so a square root transformation is needed**

—**the table does not give the mean and standard deviation of change in outcome, measured within patient on the transformed data, which are needed for paired comparison using Student's t-test**

Twenty-eight patients with chronic stable angina entered a randomised double-blind cross-over trial that compared propranolol 80 mg daily with placebo. The trial periods were two weeks each. At the end of the cross-over study all patients were put on propranolol 80 mg daily and monitored on an open basis for another four weeks, and the outcome at the end of the second fortnight was recorded. The table summarises changes in ST-segment in response to exercise, anginal attacks, and consumption of trinitrin

TABLE   Means and standard deviations: 28 patients

Observation	Randomised cross-over trial of placebo (2 weeks)		Randomised cross-over trial of propranolol (2 weeks)		Open study of propranolol (4 weeks)	
	mean	SD	mean	SD	mean	SD
(Peak ST-segment*/ exercise time) x 1000	341	33	199	17	195	17
Anginal attacks per 2 weeks	14·1	5·3	6·7	2·8	4·0	2·2
Trinitrin (mg)per 2 weeks	19·6	5·0	9·7	3·4	4·3	2·1

*lead CM5

COMMENT

Since variance is not constant for any of the three measures of outcome the observations need to be transformed before analysis. A constant ratio of mean to standard deviation indicates a logarithmic transformation. To take response to exercise as an example, the three ratios are similar, being $341/33 = 10·3$; $199/17 = 11·7$; $195/17 = 11·5$. A constant ratio of mean to variance on the other hand shows the need for square root transformation as in the case of trinitrin dose, the ratios of mean to variance being $19·6/25·0 = 0·8$; $9·7/11·6 = 0·8$; $4·3/4·4 = 1·0$. Having obtained as transformed observations for each patient the logarithm of response to exercise, the logarithm of the number of anginal attacks, and the square root of trinitrin dose, the investigator should then check that variance is approximately constant on the transformed scales and that the distribution of within-patient differences (placebo versus propranolol) is approximately Gaussian. Only then should he appeal to Student's t-test to assess whether the mean difference deviates significantly from zero. Because it is mean *within-patient difference* which is being tested, the standard deviation which is relevant is the standard deviation of those differences. In addition to the table given the author should report mean within-patient differences on the transformed scales and the corresponding measures of dispersion.

Notice that the within-patient comparison of placebo versus propranolol (four weeks) is a non-randomised comparison and that patients were probably aware of being given propranolol during the open phase of the study. This knowledge may have conditioned their reporting of the frequency of anginal attacks and the dose of trinitrin used.

(30) *"Nepalese hillmen use the right hand to eat food; the food contains possibly protective herbs. Among these people, skin cancers were located significantly more often on the left hand than on the right, and so it follows that the herbs are protective against skin cancers." Comment.*

—**the conclusion does not follow from the evidence**

—**skin cancers may be more common on the left hand anyway, irrespective of eating habit**

—**even if left predominance were peculiar to the Nepalese, the herbal hypothesis is not established; a direct test of it could be made, however**

COMMENT

The conclusion does not follow from the evidence for two main reasons. Firstly, skin cancers may be more common on the left hand anyway, so that left predominance is not peculiar to the Nepalese. Secondly, even if left predominance were exaggerated in the Nepalese hillmen relative to other peoples whose diet or eating habit, or both, is different, the herbal hypothesis would not be firmly established. Other explanations come readily to mind. Beware of speculative inference. A direct test—of whether the handling of food that contains certain herbs protects against skin cancer—might be impracticable. It would at least entail long-term follow-up of subjects who had been randomised to particular combinations of diet (including or excluding certain herbs) and eating habit (use left hand, right hand, knife and fork). Comparing the incidence and time to appearance of skin cancers would be appropriate.

I gladly record my thanks to Dr Ian Sutherland, director, MRC Biostatistics Unit, and to Professor Calbert I Phillips, Department of Ophthalmology, University of Edinburgh, for constructive criticism of all of these articles.

I am grateful to Dr Stuart J Pocock, Royal Free Hospital, London, Dr Tony L Johnson, Ms Helen Tate, and Mr Derek Lowe, MRC Biostatistics Unit, for valuable commentary on particular articles, and to the many research workers who generously allowed me to reproduce figures.

I am indebted to Sue Burkhart, staff editor on the BMJ, who liaised with me in co-ordinating the series, and outlawed as many unhelpful statistical terms as was possible. The challenge of devising a suitable layout for a question and answer series was willingly and, I think, admirably met by the editorial staff of the BMJ in collaboration with Mr Derek Virtue, their medical artist, whom I thank.

Miss Sally Stephenson and Mrs Beryl Smith, MRC Biostatistics Unit, ensured the smooth preparation of these articles by the efficiency and patience of their secretarial help.

References

[1] Gore SM, Jones IG, Rytter EC. Misuse of statistical methods: critical assessment of articles in BMJ from January to March 1976. Br Med J 1977;i:85-7.

[2] Christie D. Before-and-after comparisons: a cautionary tale. Br Med J 1979;ii:85-7.

ASSESSING METHODS— STATISTICAL DISTRIBUTIONS

The importance of the Gaussian (normal) distribution derives from ties with some other commonly reported statistical distributions. The links are explained graphically not rigorously; a persistent theme is that adequate sample size and near symmetry justify an appeal to classic methods. Avoid small samples; plot the frequency distribution of your data; beware of skewness.

(1) *The chance that a random observation from Student's t distribution with 40 degrees of freedom will exceed 2·7 is 1 in 200, or $\frac{1}{2}\%$. What chance is there that a standard normal deviate exceeds 2·7?*

—from statistical tables for the normal distribution we find that the chance is less, namely 0·35%

COMMENT

The family of t distributions is indexed by n, the degrees of freedom; all are symmetrical; mean, median, and mode coincide at 0 as for the standard normal distribution (mean 0 and variance 1). The first difference between the family of Student's t distributions and the Gaussian form is that the variance of Student's t distribution with n degrees of freedom is $n/(n-2)$, provided n is an integer greater than 2. This variance exceeds 1, and so more observations are located in the tails—outside the interval from -2 to $+2$, for example—than is the case for the standard normal distribution. But notice that as the degrees of freedom increase the variance $n/(n-2)$ decreases towards 1: when n is 12, 32, 52, 102, variance of the corresponding Student's t distribution is 1·20, 1·07, 1·04, 1·02. As degrees of freedom increase not only variance but also the shape of Student's t distribution approaches the form of the Gaussian distribution with mean 0 and variance 1. This is well illustrated by Armitage.[1]

In practice Student's t distribution is familiar as the test statistic used to compare means between small random samples of observations from two normal distributions with common unknown variance, estimated from the data. It is intuitive that estimating variance from the data introduces more uncertainty the smaller the sample sizes are; the degrees of freedom indicate how wide the tails of the relevant Student's t distribution are relative to the standard normal, which would be appropriate if the population variance were reliably known.

(2) *Which of the binomial distributions in figure 1 are symmetrical or nearly symmetrical?*

—the binomial distribution is symmetrical when p, the probability of success, equals $\frac{1}{2}$

—in addition, when p is not equal to $\frac{1}{2}$: the binomial distribution is nearly symmetrical if the number of trials n is large; from figure 1 note that the distribution with p=0·8 tends to symmetry for n=30 and more so

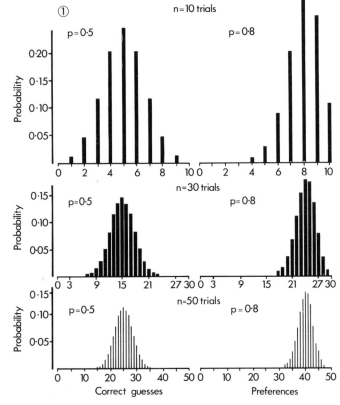

Binomial distributions: skewed if p=0·5 and n is small.

when n=50; the distribution of the number of preferences in 10 trials is quite skewed, however

COMMENT

Dinitrochlorobenzene (DNCB) dissolved in acetone was applied to one side of the head, the other side serving as control area, in 43 patients with alopecia areata.[2] The design of this study has been discussed (see page 33).[3] If it is reasonable to assume that each of the 43 patients independently has an equal chance of responding to DNCB then the number of patients in whom response favours the side treated with DNCB will have a binomial distribution with parameters n=43 (trial size) and p=probability that hair growth is more dense on the treated side. If we guess that p=0·8 then we expect to observe np=34·4 preferences for DNCB. The distribution of the number of recorded preferences would be as in figure 2. Happle and Echternacht[2] observed 33 preferences. The assumption that every patient has the same chance of responding to DNCB may not be appropriate—for example, response may depend on the extent of hair loss (moderate, extensive, total) or on how long the patient has had alopecia areata—in which case a binomial model would oversimplify the problem.

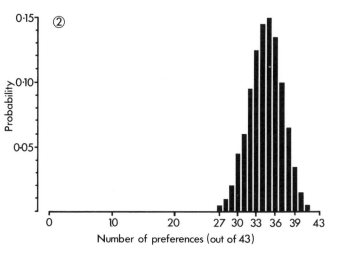

Distribution of recorded preferences: p = 0·8, n = 43, binomial.

The binomial model fits well the data reported by Elwood and Coldman[4] on the sex of children whose mothers were diagnosed as having primary breast cancer. Among 1698 children there were 851 boys, so that the probability of a child being a boy is estimated as 0·5. Table I shows the observed number of boys in families of one, two, three, and four children, and the number of boys expected according to the appropriate binomial model in which the probability of the child being a boy is estimated as 0·5. There is good agreement between observed and expected frequencies. A second example of a binomial random variable is the number of surgeons out of a total of 30, say, who, having been randomised to receive oxprenolol or placebo as matched tablets, guess correctly whether or not they have taken a beta-blocker. If oxprenolol is indistinguishable from placebo we expect 15 correct answers. Figure 1 shows that the binomial distribution is symmetrical when p = ½. For p = 0·8, the distribution is negatively skewed for small n; in the case that p is not equal to ½, the coefficient of skewness vanishes only as n—the sample size—increases, allowing the binomial distribution to be approximated by a Gaussian distribution with mean np and variance np(1−p). The approximation is adequate provided that both np and n(1−p) exceed five and is convenient because it avoids laborious summation of binomial probabilities. Notice, however, that a discrete random variable—the number of preferences for DNCB, the number of correct guesses—is approximated by a continuous one.

(3) *From the expected Poisson counts in tables II and III what do you infer about the shape of the distribution if the Poisson rate λ is low?*

—**the Poisson distribution shows strongly positive skewness for small λ**

—**if the mean count exceeds five then the Poisson distribution is more nearly symmetrical, and closer to the Gaussian form**

TABLE II—*Cases of acute poisoning on 49 purnima days*

	Number of admissions					Total
	0	1	2	3	≥4	
Observed frequency	16	23	8	2	0	49
Expected frequency (Poisson with rate λ = 0·92)	19·6	18·0	8·2	2·5	0·7	49

TABLE III—*Cases of acute poisoning on 1412 non-purnima days*

	Number of admissions					Total
	0	1	2	3	≥4	
Observed frequency	836	419	109	33	15	1412
Expected frequency (Poisson with rate λ = 0·56)	803·5	453·0	127·7	24·0	3·8	1412

COMMENT

Thakur *et al*[5] recorded the number of patients admitted with acute poisoning to Patna Medical College Hospital on each of 49 purnima days—that is, days of full moon. Forty-five people were admitted, giving a rate of (45/49) = 0·92 cases of acute poisoning per purnima day. Provided that there was no regularity in the pattern of admissions and that it was unlikely that clusters of cases would present—members of one family, for example—then the Poisson distribution with rate λ = 0·92 might describe the frequency of days on which there were no cases or one, two, three, or more cases of acute poisoning. Table II shows that the observed frequencies agree tolerably well with those expected if the number of admissions were a Poisson random variable with rate 0·92.

Patients with acute poisoning on 1412 non-purnima days—also reported by Thakur—were admitted at a rate of (796/1412) = 0·56 per non-purnima day, but the observed frequencies are not consistent with Poisson counts; there was an excess both of days on which there were no admissions and of days on which there were multiple admissions (see table III), suggesting some clustering of cases or variation in λ from day to day.

The distribution of Poisson counts is highly skewed when λ—the rate or intensity of events—is low, as in tables II and III. Approximation by a Gaussian distribution with mean and variance equal to λ is inadequate unless λ, the mean count, is high enough for this skewness to have been mostly overcome. The figure suggests that if λ exceeds five the distribution of Poisson counts is more nearly symmetrical and closer to the Gaussian form.

When comparing observed and expected counts in a two-way table, investigators are habitually warned that care is needed if an expected frequency is less than five. Why five? The explanation is implicit in the figure—the distribution of Poisson counts

TABLE I—*Number of sons in the families of women with primary breast cancer*

	Family size													
	1		2			3				4				
No of boys	0	1	0	1	2	0	1	2	3	0	1	2	3	4
Observed frequency	93	71	65	134	83	26	71	75	26	11	21	30	28	4
Expected frequency	82	82	70·5	141	70·5	24·8	74·2	74·2	24·8	5·9	23·5	35·3	23·5	5·9

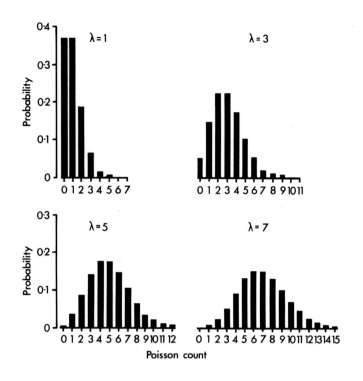

Poisson distributions: positively skewed if λ, Poisson mean, is small.

being approximately normal if the mean or expected count exceeds five and the contribution $(O-E)^2/E$ being then like the square of a standard normal deviate (see table IV).

References

[1] Armitage P. The t distribution. *Statistical methods in medical research.* Oxford: Blackwell Scientific, 1977.
[2] Happle R, Echternacht K. Induction of hair growth in alopecia areata with DNCB. *Lancet* 1977;ii:1002-3.
[3] Gore SM. Assessing clinical trials—design I. *Br Med J* 1981;**282**:1780-1.
[4] Elwood M, Coldman A. Age of mothers with breast cancer and sex of their children. *Br Med J* 1981;**282**:734.
[5] Thakur CP, Sharma RN, Akhtar HSMQ. Full moon and poisoning. *Br Med J* 1980;**281**:1684.

This was not published in the original series.

TABLE IV—*Statistical distributions and their ties to the Gaussian (normal) family*

Distribution	linked	(reason)	to
(1) Student's t distribution with n degrees of freedom	as degrees of freedom increase	variance decreases to 1	normal (Gaussian) distribution with mean 0 and variance 1
(2) Binomial distribution with parameters p (proportion of successes) and n (number of patients)	as n increases	the coefficient of skewness vanishes	normal (Gaussian) distribution with mean np and variance np(1−p) as for the binomial
(3) Poisson distribution with rate λ: for small λ the distribution of Poisson counts is positively skewed	as λ increases	the coefficient of skewness vanishes	normal (Gaussian) distribution with mean and variance equal to λ as for the Poisson

Other links

(4) lognormal with normal distribution: serum urea has a lognormal distribution and so $\log_e$ (serum urea) is normally distributed.
(5) chi-square distribution with 1 degree of freedom and normal (Gaussian) distribution with mean 0 and variance 1: if X is a standard normal random observation then X^2 has chi-squared distribution with 1 degree of freedom.
(6) chi-squared with 1 degree of freedom and chi-squared with n degrees of freedom: the sum of n independent observations, each distributed as $\chi^2_{(1)}$, is distributed as $\chi^2_{(n)}$.
(7) from Poisson to normal and normal to chi-squared: this link is responsible for how we analyse two-way tables summing $(O-E)^2/E$ over each cell in the table. The observed count is a Poisson random variable with mean or expectation E if the null hypothesis is correct.

Index